Graham Lawton is a senior staff writer and columnist at *New Scientist* magazine and the writer behind two *New Scientist* books published by John Murray Press: *The Origin of (Almost) Everything* (2018) and *This Book Could Save Your Life: The Science of Living Longer Better* (2020).

He has a BSc in Biochemistry and an MSc in Science Communication, both from Imperial College London. He lives in London.

Also by Graham Lawton

The Origin of (Almost) Everything

This Book Could Save Your Life:
The Science of Living Longer Better

MUSTN'T GRUMBLE

The surprising science of everyday ailments
and why we're always a bit ill

GRAHAM LAWTON

First published in 2021 by Headline Home an imprint of Headline Publishing Group

First published in paperback in 2023

2

Cataloguing in Publication Data is available from the British Library

ISBN 978 1 4722 8364 1

Copy editor: Lindsay Davies
Proofreader: Jill Cole
Indexer: Caroline Wilding

Designed and typeset by EM&EN
Printed and bound in Great Britain by Clays Ltd, Elcograf S.p.A.

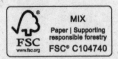

HEADLINE PUBLISHING GROUP
An Hachette UK Company
Carmelite House
50 Victoria Embankment
London EC4Y 0DZ

www.headline.co.uk
www.hachette.co.uk

This edition of *Mustn't Grumble* is dedicated to
the memory of my beloved wife Clare,
who lived a life of interesting minor ailments
but then developed a major one and died.
Her illness was called musculoskeletal nociplastic
pain syndrome, which is when the way the brain
perceives pain goes wrong, leading to constant,
excruciating agony. She fell ill in October 2021
and killed herself on 23 August 2022.

Contents

Introduction

In recent months I've been keeping a secret diary. Although its contents are a little embarrassing, I've kept it going in the name of science. I call it my 'Mustn't Grumble' book – a daily litany of all my minor ailments. I won't detain you with the slightly gruesome details, but some of the edited highlights include a mild cold, a small but painful burn on my right thumb, a blister caused by my new trainers, a twitchy eyelid that lasted three days, a bout of diarrhoea, two zits and a stubbed toe. There's also the ongoing saga of my sore shoulder and persistent athlete's foot.

My diary rarely has a break. Since I started it, not one day has gone by when I had nothing at all to enter. And I can't see one coming any time soon. Keeping a record has confirmed what I suspected – that I'm constantly ill. So are my wife and sons, and I think most of the rest of us are too. We're not hypochondriacs; we're just human, which means being a bit ill most of the time.

Which is very annoying. Like many people, I vaguely aspire to 'wellness' – that nebulous term that owes more to marketing than science. But if we define wellness as the absence of illness, then my goal is perpetually out of reach. Even more so in the strange new world in which we find ourselves. I'm writing this in autumn 2020, as the Covid-19 pandemic grinds ever onwards. One of its effects has been to make us all much more vigilant about our health in general, and minor symptoms in particular. And this, perhaps, has made us all much more conscious that we feel slightly out of sorts a great deal of the time.

Think about it: when was the last time you enjoyed a day of perfect health? A day when there was nothing – absolutely nothing – wrong with you?

I'm not talking about being *ill* ill, the kind of illness that forces you to take to your bed or make an appointment at the doctor's (good luck with that – before the pandemic they were too busy dealing with other people's minor ailments; now they're too busy dealing with major ones). I'm referring to the mild, irritating illnesses and aches and pains that we put up with all the time. And there's a lot that can go wrong. My personal diary of ailments has barely scratched the surface. I live in Britain where the National Health Service (NHS) long ago replaced the Church of England as the nation's established religion – even more so after its Covid-19 heroics. The NHS helpfully issues a leaflet listing twenty-one official minor ailments, including colds, indigestion and backache, but from my experience it's woefully incomplete. So I've made my own list, and it has nearly 100 entries.

On Christmas Day 2019, as the pandemic was brewing on the other side of the world, my wife and I went out for a walk in a local park and tried to think of any I'd missed.

'Piles?' she said.

'Yep, I've got piles,' I said.

'Worms and nits?'

'Yes, got worms and nits too. But not crabs.'

We got some very funny looks.

Minor ailments are a common topic of conversation between us – probably not the most frequent, but definitely in the top two. Again, I don't think we're unusual. Anthropologists who study small talk have found that, predictably, most social chit-chat is about the weather. But I bet if they eavesdropped on families, everyday health grumbles would win hands down. I don't know of any actual research along those lines so will offer up an anecdote instead. My sister-in-law knows a couple who have a modified swear box in their house. Unlike a normal swear box, it is designed not as a deterrent against profanity but health grumbles. Anyone caught griping about a minor ailment has to pay a fine into it. It's bulging with cash, enough to pay for an indefinite supply of over-the-counter remedies.

Many people don't stop at grumbling. Around three-quarters of family doctor appointments in the UK are for eight of what the NHS calls 'self-care conditions': back pain, dermatitis, heartburn and indigestion, blocked noses, constipation, coughs, acne and sprains. In the US, about 25 million people a year visit their doctor with uncomplicated upper respiratory infections, a.k.a. common colds. The NHS is so fed up with people taking up doctors' precious time with trivial complaints that it is training support staff – nurses, paramedics, medical assistants and pharmacists – to deal with them.

It's worth noting at this point that there's no scientific, medical or even legal definition of a minor ailment. As a rule of thumb, they are illnesses that resolve themselves or can be cured without heavy-duty medical intervention. But not always. Minor does not necessarily mean trivial. For some people — for example, those with a weakened immune system — minor ailments can progress to something much worse. Some are early symptoms of a more serious disease. So don't assume that this book dismisses minor ailments. I've tried to keep the tone light, but it's not always possible to draw a clear and distinct line.

It's also worth noting that I'm a science writer, not a doctor* and thus not qualified to dispense personal medical advice.

---

* I often need to remind my wife of this. Since I started writing this book, she has treated me like her personal physician. I keep on telling her that even though I know a lot about minor ailments in general, I do not know about her minor ailments in particular, and can neither diagnose what ails her nor recommend a course of treatment. This is the difference between a scientist and a doctor.

If you have a minor ailment that is affecting your quality of life, getting worse or otherwise troubling you, ignore me and go and see a medical professional.

Nonetheless, we usually regard minor ailments as little more than what doctors would call a *cervicalgia* – a pain in the neck. But I think they deserve more attention and respect.

Human biology is a fascinating subject, and one in which we all have a great personal interest. We can learn a lot about it from when things go a bit wrong. Consider one of the working titles of this book, *Warts and All*.* To understand warts requires a grasp of virology, genetics, immunology, anatomy and stem-cell biology, plus some knowledge of folklore and history. Knowing a little more about minor ailments should also help us to get better faster – or even avoid them in the first place.

Arguably they even deserve our gratitude. Victorious Roman generals employed slaves to whisper *memento mori* ('remember that you will die') in their ears during their victory parades, to keep them from resting on their laurels. This is how I see minor ailments: a constant, nagging reminder that we're mortal, but that it could be worse, and one day it will be. So, mustn't grumble. After all, what doesn't kill you only makes you stronger.

---

* I also considered calling it *What Doesn't Kill You* . . . but I know from previous experience that publishers do not like book titles with words such as 'kill' and 'death' in them. My previous book is called *This Book Could Save Your Life*, which is all about prolonging lifespan and healthspan through health and fitness. I wanted to call it *This Book Could Postpone Your Death*, which I argued was more attention-grabbing and also more honest. The publisher did not agree.

1
OUCH!

Being in pain is no fun, but we'd miss it if it wasn't there. It is nature's way of telling us to back off. Pain is a reliable signal that we are injured or ill and a motivator to take immediate remedial action. To mangle a well-known phrase, if something's hurting, it ain't working.

Next time you are in pain, take comfort from the fact that it doesn't really exist. Like the experience of seeing colour, it is merely an illusion created by the brain to help us negotiate our way through life and keep it going as long as possible.

Pain is produced by specialist nerve endings called nociceptors that are distributed throughout the body, though not in the brain. When they detect a potential threat such as an injury, they send a warning signal to the spinal cord, which relays it to a region of the midbrain called the thalamus for analysis. If the threat is judged to be credible, the thalamus sends a message back to where the signal came from ordering it to hurt, and a memo to the cerebral cortex to create conscious awareness of the pain.

The experience of pain varies, both in intensity and quality. There is no way of objectively measuring either, so we have to take people's word for it. There are dozens of subjective pain scales, often numbered from one to ten, with one being 'no pain' and ten being 'the worst possible pain'.

The quality of pain correlates somewhat with its intensity, but not completely. One widely used pain quality assessment asks about intensity but also to what extent that pain is stabbing, hot, dull, sensitive, tender, shooting, tingling, numb, throbbing and more. It also asks whether the pain is deep or surface. These differences are largely determined by which type of nerve fibres are damaged. Damage to pain or temperature receptors produces sharp, stabby, hot pain, whereas damage to touch receptors produces a duller numbness. Location matters too: musculoskeletal pain is often deep, dull and achy, whereas pain from an injury is sharp and on the surface.

Throbbing is widely assumed to be caused by the pulsing of blood to the site of an injury, but that's not what's happening. As a rule, the rate of throbbing is slower than the pulse and there is no synchrony between the two. The experience of throbbing is probably a subjective sensation created by the brain as part of the general pain experience. What, if any, purpose it serves beyond making the pain even more unpleasant is not known.

Whatever its subjective quality, pain is unpleasant, and for good reason. It is a powerful and immediate motivator to withdraw from whatever is hurting us, to protect and nurture a damaged body part to give it time to heal, and to avoid similar situations in future. It thus enhances survival, and so was selected by evolution. It is literally the opposite of pleasure. Just as pleasurable sensations motivate us to seek out survival-enhancing stimuli such as food and sex, painful ones motivate us to avoid survival-limiting ones.

To understand the biological utility of pain, consider people with the rare genetic disorder called congenital analgesia, which means they cannot feel pain. People who have it must learn to be extremely vigilant in their daily lives to avoid seriously injuring themselves. Even something as mundane as drinking a hot drink is fraught with danger. People with the condition usually die young from unnoticed injuries or infections.

So curse and grimace all you like, but also give pain credit where it's due. If it's hurting, then chances are your body is working.

My head hurts

If 'not tonight, I've got a headache' feels like a massive snub, try this one on for size: 'Stop, it's giving me a headache!'

Headaches are mysterious at the best of times, but why they can be triggered by sex is totally baffling. The 'headache associated with sexual activity'[1] usually begins alongside the stirrings of sexual arousal and builds with it, climaxing at the same time as its unfortunate sufferer. Or sometimes it strikes all at once just before or during orgasm – with a bang, so to speak. But unlike orgasms it can last for days. The intense pain can go on for twenty-four hours and linger for another forty-eight. Fortunately, the sex headache is quite rare, affecting roughly one in 100 people, mostly men. Why it happens, nobody knows.

You can pretty much say the same about all the other types of headache, of which around 200 are listed in the International Headache Society's *International Classification of Headache Disorders*.[2] It's enough to make your head hurt.

Headaches are extremely common, perhaps even more so than the common cold.[3] The vast majority are just a mysterious pain in the head rather than a sign of anything serious. Around 90 per cent of cases are of the normal, ordinary variety that almost everyone endures from time to time.

Of course, some headaches are not minor. About one in ten cases are migraines and a category called trigeminal autonomic cephalalgias (TACs), the best-known of which are cluster headaches, characterised by periodic recurrent attacks (or clusters) of severe pain on one side of the head, usually around the eye. Both types are deeply unpleasant – cluster headaches are sometimes called 'suicide headaches' because of their severity – and decidedly non-trivial, so enough of them.

Brain tumours can also cause headaches but almost always have other symptoms as well; only 1 per cent of brain tumours have headache as their only symptom. So rest assured that if your head hurts but you're otherwise okay, it probably isn't cancer.

Did I say 'if' your head hurts? Make that 'when'. Almost everyone gets a headache from time to time, with a lifetime prevalence of 96 per cent. Headaches are 'an almost universal human experience', according to a 2017 review article in the *American Journal of Medicine*.[4] And they go back a long way. The earliest-known medical description is in the Ebers Papyrus, an Ancient Egyptian medical text written in about 1550 BC, but they were almost certainly pounding human heads long before that. 'We are justified in assuming that headache has always been with *Homo sapiens*', wrote Arnold Friedman, head of the Headache Unit at Montefiore Hospital in New York back in 1972.[5]

The common ones are what neurologists call 'tension-type headaches', which erroneously suggests that they are known to be caused by tension.[6] Tension and stress have been proposed as a trigger, but according to the International Headache Society, 'the exact mechanisms . . . are not known.' Some of these headaches-without-a-cause are truly weird. The nummular headache, for example, is an intensely painful coin-sized patch on the scalp. The hypnic headache strikes during sleep; the stabbing headache is self-explanatory and the thunderclap headache is a rapid-onset, intensely painful headache often mistaken for a brain aneurism. Sex headaches sometimes arrive in thunderclap form.

There are some headaches for which underlying causes are known. These includes blows to the head, infections such as colds and sinusitis, violent coughing, caffeine withdrawal, taking too many painkillers, eating ice cream, bad teeth, hangovers and, of course, sex. Masturbation can also bring on a sex headache, making headaches one of the minor ailments that onanism – which has been unfairly blamed for all sorts of things from warts to short sightedness – can actually cause.

Among these 'secondary headaches', the hangover headache – technically called the delayed alcohol-induced headache – is among the most common. It is often attributed to dehydration but probably isn't (see page 297). As usual, the true cause remains hazy.

Ditto the ice-cream headache, or brain freeze, which I was told as a child was caused by nerves in my teeth being frozen, but which is more likely blood vessels in the palate suddenly constricting in response to cold.

There are many things that are often said to cause headaches that are not recognised in the classification system, including stress, dehydration, bad eyesight and high-pressure weather.

Even though a headache can feel like it is your brain hurting, it isn't. Brains do not have pain receptors and cannot hurt. Headaches are actually the result of pain receptors elsewhere in the head screaming out in protest at whatever is aggravating them. That includes receptors in the blood vessels and nerves surrounding the brain, in the three meningeal membranes wrapped around it, and in muscles in the face and neck. In fact, muscle pain is the leading cause of headaches and can make the head painful to the touch. But, unsurprisingly, its cause is not known.

Whatever the underlying cause, tension-type headaches are all remarkably similar. To be diagnosed as one, the pain must tick at least two boxes from a checklist of four: mild to moderate in intensity; not localised to one side of the head; not throbbing; and not worsened by routine physical activity. In addition, doctors will check there is no nausea or vomiting, and that the patient is not aversive to both bright light and loud sounds (aversion to one or the other is allowed). If the headache passes these tests it is probably nothing to worry about. If not, it could be more serious and requires further medical investigation, as there are a good many very serious causes of headaches ranging from brain haemorrhages to meningitis.

For most people, tension-type headaches are an occasional irritant, occurring less than once a month – though a single episode can last for up to a week. But some people have more frequent attacks, up to ten a month, and an unlucky few suffer from chronic headaches, which means having one most days. According to the World Health Organization, something like 5 per cent of people are in this unfortunate bind.[7] Why this happens is not known.

Even though tension-type headaches are classified as a minor ailment by the NHS, they can be debilitating. In a recent study in the *Journal of the American Medical Association*, 8 per cent of people with infrequent headaches took sick days because of them, and nearly half said they were less effective at work or school when they had a headache.[8] For people with chronic headaches the impacts are even higher.

As for treatment, 'few evidence-based guidelines exist', according to a recent review of the evidence.[9] The first line of defence is simple painkillers.

But beware: another proven cause of headaches is medication overuse, including the overuse of painkillers. Some people get into a vicious circle, taking ever more painkillers to dull the pain but just making it worse. You will not be surprised to learn that the reason for this remains unknown.

Painkillers are not the only option. There is reasonably strong evidence that applying Tiger Balm – a volatile and pungent ointment from Singapore heavily laced with menthol, eucalyptus and camphor – is better than nothing.[10]

My mother-in-law (who you will meet a lot in this book) has her own remedy: the so-called 'headache sandwich', which consists of marigold leaves squished between two pieces of buttered bread. My wife and her siblings were all served this bizarre remedy as children; one reviewer (my wife) describes them as 'horrible'. There is some method to this madness, but only some: *Calendula officinalis* leaves are edible and have mild anti-inflammatory properties, though the leaves are usually brewed into a medicinal tea, not put in a sandwich.

If headache sandwiches are not your cup of tea, you could always try tying a piece of cake to your head. Folk medicine has no shortage of headache cures which, as usual, have more entertainment than medicinal value.[11] But none is as strange as this American recipe from 1657, which instructs that 'a piece of Red Rose Cake . . . be cut fit for the Head [and] must lie next to the Forehead and Temples and bound so thereto for all night'.

Having cake strapped to your head is probably also an effective deterrent to unwanted sexual advances. Not tonight, I've got a head cake.

Aches and pains

One of the most annoying things about getting older is that things start to hurt for no apparent reason. Right now I get knee pains when I walk down the stairs. My right shoulder aches from time to time. The ball of my left foot sometimes throbs. My ankle has a tendency to click out. I often wake up in the morning with an inexplicable pain somewhere. I sometimes feel like I am falling apart at the seams.

Which is because I am. My aches and pains are all in my joints, those useful but damage-prone parts of the body where bone meets bone.

Joint pain is extremely common, especially among middle-aged and elderly people. About two-thirds of people aged sixty-five and over have one or more painful joint, and even among younger people the prevalence is about 40 per cent. There are some serious causes, including rheumatoid arthritis, cancer, bone fractures and infections. Gout is also a common, and singularly horrible, source of joint pain (see page 39). But most of the time the problem is simple wear and tear.

Knees are especially susceptible to damage as they bear so much weight – everything from the knees upwards – and have so many moving parts. The knee is the largest, most complex and hardest-working joint in the human body. Technically speaking, it is two joints, one between the thigh bone and shin bone and the other between the thigh bone and kneecap. They can both flex and rotate and are crammed full of things that can become injured or worn out – muscles, cartilages, ligaments and tendons. And as we become collectively heavier, our knees are becoming collectively more knackered.

One common cause of knee pain is tendonitis, when one or more of the tendons in the knee is injured and becomes inflamed. Tendons are straps of tough connective tissue that join muscles to bones. The main one in the knee is the patellar tendon, which connects the muscle at the front thigh to the shin bone (tibia) and straps the kneecap (patella) in place. Running, jumping and twisting can damage it and cause it to become inflamed, leading to pain between the kneecap and shin. Rest, ice packs, painkillers and a support bandage will usually allow it to heal naturally.

The ligaments, which connect bone to bone, can also become inflamed or torn. Knees contain four major ones, including the two cruciate ligaments that are often the location of severe and sometimes career-ending injuries for footballers. When the fiery Manchester United midfielder Roy Keane 'did' his cruciate in a game against Leeds United in 1997, he says he actually heard it snap.

It takes extreme force to snap a knee ligament, but over-stretching and minor tears are not uncommon. Ligament damage is one of the most frequent sources of knee pain; not only does it hurt a lot but it can also lead to swelling, restricted movement and wobbly knees that can give way at the drop of a hat. But as with tendon damage, rest and support bandages are a great healer, though reconstructive surgery of the kind that saved Keane's career is occasionally necessary.

Damage to the knee cartilage – a tough but flexible tissue that coats the ends of bones to cushion and lubricate the points where they meet – is similarly career-threatening for athletes. Ordinary people can damage their cartilages too, leading to pain, swelling, stiffness, knee instability or locking and a sickening clicking or grinding noise when the knee moves. This is in fact exactly what's happening – the ends of the bones are grinding directly against one another. The cartilage underneath the kneecap is especially prone to damage through overuse; this is called 'runner's knee', for good reason. The pain is often worse when moving but can hurt when at rest. Again, cartilage damage will usually resolve itself with a bit of TLC but may eventually require surgery or even a bionic replacement.

As with knees, so with other joints: hips, ankles, shoulders, elbows, fingers, necks and toes. All are complex and hard-working contraptions of bone, muscle, ligament, tendon and cartilage, and can be injured in all sorts of interesting ways.

Ankles often do something that other joints don't: click and pop. There are two main reasons for this, neither of which is any great cause for concern.

One is the release of dissolved gases from the joint capsule, a bag of goo called synovial fluid which helps to lubricate the joint. When the joint is inactive, gases such as nitrogen can dissolve into the fluid; when it springs into action, such as when you leap out of bed in the morning, the fluid is compressed, the nitrogen un-dissolves and turns back into a gas, forming bubbles which pop noisily. This is also what causes knuckles to crack. Regardless of what you have heard, it is not damaging to the joints and does not lead to arthritis.

The other common cause of clicky ankles is slipped tendons. Two of the tendons connecting the calf muscles to the bones of the foot run along a groove at the back of the ankle. The groove is a bit too wide and the tendons can slip slightly out of place. That is what leads to the sensation – again, often first thing in the morning or after a long sit down – that the ankle has clicked out of place. It has. But it will easily click back in, with a satisfying sound and no lasting damage.

Cartilage can also just wear out, a condition called osteo-arthritis (arthritis is a catch-all term for inflammation of the joints; *osteo* is Greek for bone). Over time, the protective cushion is gradually eroded away and daily use becomes a daily grind. Osteoarthritic joints – especially the long-suffering knees but also hips and fingers – become painful and stiff and can emit a grating noise when moving.

The symptoms vary from person to person and from day to day, but tend to intensify after exercise and worsen over time. It is usually most painful first thing in the morning, which can make going downstairs a daily feat of endurance.

The main risk factor is age. Osteoarthritis is literally your joints wearing out. It is an occupational hazard of being alive, especially if you are active: minor joint injuries from running or playing sports can progress to osteoarthritis if they are not given time to heal, an irony that is not lost on me and my poor knees, which I fear I have irreparably damaged by forcing them to carry my ever-increasing body weight on regular pavement-pounding runs.

Osteoarthritis can't be cured. But it can be eased by low-impact exercise, sensible shoes and support bandages or walking sticks. Which, like the pain that necessitates them, are among the joys of getting old.

Another joint that is very prone to painful and debilitating injury is the shoulder. This problem is often located in the rotator cuff, a cluster of muscles and tendons surrounding the ball-and-socket joint that connects the shoulder blade to the upper arm. The muscles of the cuff are key enablers of the huge range of movement – nearly full 360-degree rotation – of which the human shoulder is capable. This makes us uniquely good at overarm throwing, which probably contributed to our evolutionary success by enabling our ancestors to throw spears at woolly mammoths.

But it means that the rotator cuff is an intricate bit of kit that can become injured or worn out in myriad ways. The cuff also stabilises the joint, which is quite ill-fitting as the ball is slightly too big for the socket.

Repetitive movements such as using a computer mouse or stacking shelves can irritate tendons or cause certain muscles to weaken through under-use. A cuff injury can progress to adhesive capsulitis, commonly and aptly called frozen shoulder. Without treatment, shoulder pain can last for years. Physiotherapy can usually help, but avoid the temptation to come up with your own exercise regime. A qualified physio needs to assess the shoulder, work out exactly what is wrong and prescribe appropriate exercises. The wrong ones can just make it worse.

The anthropologist and TV presenter Alice Roberts is a world expert on rotator cuff injuries in humans and other apes; she wrote her PhD thesis on them and discovered that pretty much everyone, human and ape alike, develops a bad shoulder in the end. Eventually, we all just fall apart at the seams.

Muscle knots

'Where does it hurt?' might seem like an obvious and useful question to ask somebody who is in pain. The answer, however, can be painfully wide of the mark. Unless the source of pain is an injury, it may well be a manifestation of a problem a long way from where it actually hurts.

That problem is often a muscle knot, technically called a myofascial trigger point. These common but controversial little lumps of misery are a frequent source of pain elsewhere, almost as if they want to keep their presence a secret.

Back pain, for example, often originates from a muscle knot in the abdominals – literally on the opposite side of the torso. Headaches can originate in the neck (see page 11), leg pain in the buttocks and ankle pain in the calf. Knots in a shoulder muscle can send pain right down the arms and into the hands. Unexplained toothache and earache have also been traced back to muscle knots. The knots can also restrict movement in the muscle, so are a leading cause of cricked neck (see page 23).

This 'referred pain' may be why so many aches and pains have no apparent cause and end up being diagnosed as non-specific. About 80 per cent of cases of back pain, for example, are chucked into this medical wastebasket and not investigated further.

Myofascial trigger points are essentially cramps that don't involve the whole muscle (see page 302). They happen when, for various reasons, small patches of muscle tissue become hyper-sensitive.

The word 'myofascial' refers to the dense connective tissue that wraps around skeletal muscles. Anatomically speaking, a myofascial trigger point is a tender patch of muscle tissue about halfway along a band of unusually taut muscle fibres. To the touch, they feel like a hard or squelchy nodule just under the skin. Although commonly found in the back, neck and shoulders, they can arise anywhere in skeletal muscles – the ones we voluntarily contract to move our bodies rather than the involuntary ones in internal organs.

Touching them can trigger local and/or referred pain and also cause a tell-tale twitch of the taut band as its trigger-happy muscle fibres briefly contract.

The hard-yet-squelchy feeling of a muscle knot, and the fact that massaging them with fingertips can 'break them up' (often causing weirdly pleasurable discomfort not unlike the sensation of a banged funny bone) has led to a belief that they are an accumulation of lactic acid crystals. They are not. Massage works by encouraging the cramped-up muscle fibres to relax, which causes the knot to shrink and even vanish, along with the pain. The relief can be considerable.

Knots can also be alleviated with alternating cold and hot compresses, which reduce any swelling and encourage the knot to relax itself. Rest, stretching and gentle exercise can also help, but there is little evidence that rubs such as Tiger Balm, Deep Heat and wintergreen – collectively called rubefacients – relax muscle knots. However, they may relieve pain through a rather vague and unproven mechanism called counterirritation, which is the medicinal equivalent of stamping on somebody's foot to take their mind off a punch to the nose. The preparations contain irritant compounds such as menthol, camphor, capsaicin and clove oil, which rub the skin up the wrong way and can desensitise it to other sources of pain, in part by causing the sensory neurons to fire to the point of exhaustion. Or so the theory goes. The UK's National Institute for Health and Care Excellence (NICE), which is basically the NHS's penny pincher, says there is not enough evidence to support their use.

Some rubs also contain compounds called salicylates,

which are related to aspirin, and it is often claimed that these are absorbed into the skin and can kill the pain. But again there is no evidence that this is true. But the irritant rubs can be paradoxically soothing and won't do any harm, so rub yourself out.

There are also painkilling muscle rubs containing ibuprofen and paracetamol, but these are no more effective than swallowing tablets and take longer to kick in: up to a day compared with less than an hour. And they should not be used to top up the painkilling if you have already taken the maximum daily oral dose: the drugs still find their way into the bloodstream and count towards the total.

Really bad knots may need injections of anaesthetic, anti-inflammatories or even Botox to relieve the pain.

Muscle knots are very common, possibly the most common cause of musculoskeletal pain. One study of patients in a specialist pain clinic found that 85 per cent of them had one or more myofascial trigger points. The renowned Czech doctor Karl Lewit went further and proposed in 2009 that they are the most common cause of pain, period. Yet doctors often do not even consider them when investigating otherwise-unexplained pain.

One reason for this medical blind spot is that they have become tainted by association with acupuncture, chiropractic and other alternative medical practices. This is a shame. Some doctors argue that an awful lot of pain and discomfort could be avoided or resolved if trigger points were taken more seriously by mainstream medicine.

Another problem is that there is no agreed cause of myofascial trigger points, nor of referred pain. Formation of trigger points is associated with all sorts of things, including poor posture, overuse or overstretching of a muscle (a hazard of failing to warm up before exercise), and inactivity. Dehydration, smoking, poor diet and stress have also been linked to their formation.

Referred pain, meanwhile, clearly has something to do

with sensory nerve fibres radiating pain signals away from their source to another part of the body. A muscle knot in one place predictably causes pain in another, not in some random body part. But the exact mechanism is unknown.

If you have unexplained pain somewhere in your body – the pain is usually described as deep but somewhat diffuse – it is worth having a dig around for a squelchy lump somewhere else. It's no wonder myofascial trigger points are so common: humans have approximately 640 skeletal muscles which typically account for 40 to 50 per cent of body weight. For bodybuilders, it can be as much as 65 per cent. That is a lot of muscle to get knotted.

Cricked neck

Most minor ailments are annoying, but only a select few are *so* annoying that their names have become bywords for 'annoying'. One is a pain in the arse (see page 214). The other is a pain in the neck.

Neck pain is nature's way of reminding you how useful it is to be able to turn your head. We've all endured a day or three of pain and stiffness that forces us to turn our entire bodies just to look at things, like a zombie. It can make everyday activities such as driving and cycling almost impossible.

There are various causes of what is commonly known as cricked neck or wry neck. Sleeping or sitting in a draught is not one of them, unless the draught causes you to hold your head in a strange and unnatural posture for a prolonged period of time, which can lead to muscle stiffness exactly like that caused by exercising (see page 304). This is quite hard to do while awake, but easy during sleep, which is why you can go to bed in perfect neck health and wake up barely able to move it at all.

Another cause is minor strains and sprains from unnatural or extreme head movements. The terms 'strain' and 'sprain' are often used interchangeably but actually refer to different types of injury. Strains are tears to muscles and tendons; sprains are injuries to ligaments, the fibrous tissues connecting bone to bone. From the perspective of the owner of a cricked neck, however, this is splitting hairs. They can be equally painful and restrictive.

The neck is a very muscly and active part of the body – hence the aggravation when you can't move it freely – and also contains seven vertebrae, so strains and sprains have a lot of opportunities to work their mischief.

Three muscles in particular are prone to being strained on account of their large size and pivotal role in head movement. One is the trapezius, a kite-shaped muscle that connects the base of the skull to the shoulder blades and lower back and is key to extending the neck. The others are involved in head rotation: the levator scapulae, which run down each side of the neck, and the sternocleidomastoid muscles, which run from behind the ear down to the breastbone.

A bad strain in any of these muscles can lead to a visibly unusual posture, such as having the head tilted to one side or forwards. This is known as torticollis, Latin for 'twisted neck'.

Cricked neck can also be caused by muscle knots, or myofascial trigger points (see page 19).

If you do wake up with a crick in your neck, there's not a lot you can do except wait for it to get better. Painkillers can help, as can heat (which reduces muscle spasms) or cold (which dials down inflammation). A gentle massage or stretching session might ease it too. But time is the only real healer.

If the crick persists or is getting worse, go and see a doctor. Chronic cricked necks are sometimes caused by something worse than a minor injury, including trapped nerves, slipped discs and whiplash. Meningitis can also cause a stiff neck but usually has other symptoms too (see page 66).

A non-serious crick usually clears up by itself in a few days. But those days are truly a pain in the neck.

Banged funny bone

The Germans call it *der Musikantenknochen* (musician's bone). In Spain it is *hueso de la risa* (bone of laughter). Finns call it *kiukkusuoni* (anger vessel) and Hungarians *villanyozó ín* (electrifying tendon). But English surely has the best name for it: the funny bone.

People the world over know and yet struggle to describe the strange and unique sensation that comes from hitting this bit of the elbow: a mixture of tingly pain and numbness, like an electric shock, surging down the lower arm. If you give it a really good clonk the sensation can linger for several minutes. The natural response is to shake it out, often while cursing loudly, but there's no evidence that this does anything other than distract from the pain.

That vulnerable spot isn't in fact a bone at all, but an exposed bit of the nervous system called the ulnar nerve which runs from the spinal cord down the arm to the fourth and fifth fingers. As it passes through the elbow region it briefly runs close to the surface, where it is relatively unshielded by skin, bone, fat and muscle. This weak spot is called the cubital tunnel, which you can feel by probing the back of your elbow just above the joint. If you strike this bit of your anatomy on a protruding object – such as the bracket in my shower which appears perfectly positioned for it – it causes the nerve to fire.

'Funny bone' may be a play on humerus, the name of the upper arm bone that runs from the shoulder to the elbow. Or it may just be a description of the feeling when you hit it.

Striking your funny bone is harmless, but the cubital tunnel is susceptible to injuries, repetitive strain damage and trapped nerves, which can lead to cubital tunnel syndrome. This has been described as a permanent state of funny-bone pain, which is nobody's idea of fun.

My feet are killing me

The human foot is a precision instrument, beautifully designed to support our unusual style of walking and also our evolved aptitude for long-distance running. From heel to toes, every bit does its job in a coordinated dance of biology and physics. The heel is a shock absorber that bears the brunt of the impact of the foot striking the ground; the arch is like a spring which absorbs the heel impact and passes it forward to the ball of the foot to assist with the next step. The toes provide adaptable balance, plus grip and leverage. A single foot contains twenty-six bones and more than 100 muscles, ligaments and tendons. No wonder some people fetishise them.

But as with all complex machines, there's a lot that can go wrong. Our feet can kill us in all sorts of ways.

A leading reason why they go wrong is that we evolved to walk and run barefoot, but these days we generally force our feet into shoes (also a cause of athlete's foot, see page 254). People who have spent a life without shoes have wide, strong and healthy feet with extremely tough skin on the underside. In comparison, shoe-bound feet are narrow, soft-bottomed and sickly.

One common complaint in shoe-wearing countries is fallen arches, or flat feet. This is where the rigid-but-flexible arch partially or completely collapses and the whole of the bottom of the foot slumps to the ground, as if the foot has somehow deflated. Up to 30 per cent of people have one or more (two, as a rule) flat feet.

Flat feet were historically viewed as a disability. For much of the twentieth century the flat-footed were often assumed to be useless at marching and standing to attention and were excluded from military service, no doubt to their considerable relief. This was largely a cost-saving exercise as recruiting, training and then having to discharge a soldier on medical grounds expended a great sum of money. In 1923 alone, the British Army discharged 190 men on the grounds of flat feet, wasting about £10,000 in the process, worth more than half a million in today's money.

But after the Second World War, research by the army found that flat-footedness was actually no hindrance to being a good soldier, and by the time of the Vietnam War, flat-footed soldiers were tramping flat-footedly (and disgruntledly) all over South-East Asia.

A few cases of flat-footedness (also called pes planus, which is Latin for 'foot flat') cause secondary problems with posture or gait but, on the whole, being flat of foot is entirely harmless. The cause is not well understood, though being obese is a clear risk factor. The arch literally collapses under its own body weight.

Another foot condition that can exempt its (un)fortunate victim from military service is heel spurs. These are small, painful, bony outgrowths from the heel bone caused by repeated stress or damage, such as wearing not very sensible shoes or being obese. They are also what got a certain Donald J. Trump exempted from joining his flat-footed brethren in Vietnam in 1968.

To be fair to Trump, he was quite sporty back in the late sixties. He was the *best* baseball player in New York at the time, according to Donald J. Trump. So maybe he overdid the baseball a bit, and got himself a heel spur. It cleared up, as bone spurs generally don't. But he eventually did military service with four years as Commander-in-Chief. So give the guy a break, already, okay?

The heel, arch and other parts of the feet can also become inflamed by overuse, such as walking or running a very long way or standing up for ages. Hard surfaces, ill-fitting shoes and excess weight from a rucksack or fat belly make it worse.

This painful condition is technically called plantar fasciitis, which means inflammation of the connective tissue on the bottom of the foot, but it is commonly known as 'my-bloody-feet-are-killing-me'. Sticking them in a bucket of cold water may bring down the inflammation, or at the very least render them numb. Rest and recuperation will do the remainder.

Tight shoes can also cause bunions, which are bony and often painful lumps that grow on the side of the feet below the big toe joint. The word 'bunion' is sometimes assumed to be related to 'onion', as the lump can look like the surface of an onion breaking through the soil, but is actually derived from various Germanic words meaning 'lump'. Once bunions form, the only way to get rid of them is surgery.

Ingrowing toenails have also been linked to tight shoes. They are exactly what the name suggests – the toenail dives downward and grows painfully into the fleshy part of the toe at the side of the nail. Cutting toenails too hard can also encourage them to take revenge in this way. The first-line treatment is to soak the offending foot in warm water three or four times a day, which softens the skin around the nail and sometimes allows the nail to free itself. If that fails, it's off to the doctor for some radical clipping.

On the subject of toes, big ones are highly susceptible to being painfully banged. This is simply because they are the most sticky-out part of the foot, and people are clumsy. A stubbed toe can be very painful and can lead to spraining or straining of the ligaments or even a broken bone, in which case it requires treatment. But usually a good swear is all you need.

Intense foot pain can also be triggered by gout, but that is another story (see page 39).

One type of foot pain you really do not want is the cracked heel. The skin on the sole of the foot is very thick, in part to be a good shock absorber. But it does not have the moisturising sebaceous glands found in skin elsewhere (other than the palms of the hands) and so is prone to dehydration. That usually doesn't matter as the upper layer of dead skin is very spongy and can absorb three times its own weight in water. But if water content drops to 10 per cent or less that skin becomes rigid and cracks. The shock of having cracked skin can make walking excruciating. That really is a killer.

Motes

As a wearer of old-fashioned contact lenses, I'm horribly familiar with the discomfort of getting something in my eye. Sharp pain, instant waterworks and a frantic fingertip rummage in the eye ensue. If, as seems to happen all the time, the mote has worked its way behind the lens there is no option but to remove it. I have lost countless contact lenses after popping one out in windy conditions.

Even people who don't wear lenses are vulnerable to things in the eye. The surface of the cornea and the linings of the lids are very sensitive – vision is a precious resource and the eyes have a hair-trigger early-warning system – and even a speck of dust can feel like a lump of gritstone. Clothing fibres, eyelashes and windblown debris all seem magnetically attracted to the surface of the eye. Smoke, obviously, gets in your eyes. And if you rinse your hair without due care and attention, shampoo does too, though nobody ever wrote a song about that.

Using power tools such as drills, saws and rotavators obviously increases the risk of flying debris striking the eye at high speed, which can injure or even pierce the cornea. Wear goggles. The same applies if using caustic chemicals to, say, unblock a drain or clean the inside of an oven.

But how to remove a mote, or even some shampoo? The flood of tears from the tear ducts is usually enough to flush it out, or into the corner of the eye from where it can be removed with a fingertip. But sometimes the offending object gets lodged under the eyelid, close to the line of contact with the eyeball. That may require some additional flushing with cold, clean water; an eye bath or shower ought to do it.

Hold the eye open and rinse thoroughly. If clean water is not available, pulling the top eyelid down over the lower one can help to dislodge the foreign body. Resist the urge to rub as this can cause an abrasive intruder to scratch the surface of the cornea, which will make it feel like there is something in your eye until it heals.

The word 'mote', incidentally, is derived from a medieval Germanic word for sawdust, which was presumably a common speck to get in the eye in medieval times. Mote is the obligatory word to use for an object in the eye thanks to the Sermon on the Mount, in which former carpenter Jesus urged people to remove beams from their own eyes before commenting on motes in their brother's. Sermonise about what you know.

Another common thing-in-the-eye is rheum, also known as sleep, eye boogers or, in my house at least, custard corners. This is the yellowish sticky or crusty substance that is found in the corner of the eye upon waking up. It is a mixture of mucus, oil, tears, dead skin and other gubbins that builds up when eyes are closed for long periods. During wakefulness, blinking sweeps this mixture into the nasolacrimal duct, a kind of ocular storm drain that empties into the nasal cavity. This duct, also known as the tear duct, is the small circular orifice visible on the rim of the lower eyelid near the corner of the eye. Contrary to popular belief it does not produce tears, but drains them away, which is why a runny nose often accompanies weeping. Tears are actually produced by the lacrimal glands embedded in the skin above the eyes. When blinking is suspended in sleep, the stuff just builds up, sometimes clogging the tear ducts and occasionally glueing the eyelids shut. That used to happen to me when I fell into a drunken slumber without taking out my contact lenses. Once unglued, however, I had the very unusual experience (for me) of being able to see clearly immediately after waking up. A miracle!

Pins and needles

If you have ever attempted to stand up after sitting in an awkward posture for a while only to discover that your leg no longer belongs to you, then you have experienced what doctors call obdormition. The leg is numb and unresponsive and will crumple under pressure, leading to many a pratfall after tedious meetings.

This embarrassing/hilarious state of affairs is described the world over as the leg (or other body part) having 'fallen asleep'. Even doctors say this, though they do it in a fancy way. *Obdormire* means 'to fall asleep' in Latin.

The leg is not actually asleep, of course. Sleep is a state of the brain – though sleeping in a funny position can cause a limb to go to sleep. It is actually suffering from temporary paralysis due to prolonged pressure on a nerve, which causes it to fire to the point of exhaustion. There is also ischaemia, or lack of blood, due to prolonged restriction of the inbound blood vessels. Lack of blood starves the muscles of oxygen, which puts them temporarily out of action. Obdormition is especially common in Japan where people sit for ages in unnatural positions during tea ceremonies.

No harm is usually done. Un-restricting the blood vessels allows oxygenated blood to flow back in, which is called reperfusion. Sensation and movement slowly return, albeit painfully as constricted capillaries reopen – this is exactly the same process as regaining feeling in cold-numbed fingers and toes (see page 111). The sensation of a reperfusing body part is called 'pins and needles' in English, though many other languages describe it in terms of ants. The French say *'J'ai des fourmis'* (I have ants); in German it is *'Ameisenlaufen'* (ants running). In always-poetic Iceland, people get *'stjörnur í skónum'*, stars in the shoes. My younger son used to call it *'pings* and needles', which is perhaps an even better description. But the prize for creativity has to go to my friend's young daughter who, when she first experienced it, said, 'Ooh, I've got fizzy feet.'

Prolonged or chronic pins and needles can be a sign of trapped nerves, circulatory problems, shingles and worse. But you'll usually be back on your fizzy feet in a few minutes.

Backache

Back pain is the price we pay for being human. When our ancestors on the African savannah abandoned knuckle walking and stood upright, they immediately put large amounts of weight on their lower spines. This was evidently worth the trade-off: perhaps standing erect allowed them to spot distant prey or danger, or freed up the arms and hands to do something more useful. However, evolution has not had time to fully compensate, and so modern humans are plagued by aches, pains and stiffness in a region of the body that we might otherwise ignore. The back is, after all, out of sight. But sadly for millions of us, it is not out of mind.

The most common type of back pain is lumbago, defined as pain in the lower back between the base of the ribcage and the top of the legs. It can literally be a pain in the arse. The word 'lumbago' is derived from the Latin word *lumbus*, meaning 'loins', which makes it sound quite saucy. It is not. Loin in this sense is strictly anatomical, as in the lower five (lumbar) vertebrae.

Lumbago is staggeringly common. About 10 per cent of adults report living with it at any given time, and in the West around 90 per cent of people get it at some time in their lives. Like other aches and pains it becomes more common and debilitating as we age and our joints become increasingly clapped out (see page 14), but the first episode often occurs in our twenties and thirties. According to some estimates, 25 per cent of young adults visiting the doctor are there because of back pain. Recurrence is common, and usually worsens with each attack.

The underlying cause of most cases is never established,

largely because it doesn't really help to know. The lower back is a complex system of muscles, bones, tendons and ligaments and, when we are standing up, it actively supports the weight of the upper body. There are a lot of moving parts and static structures that can go wrong. Doctors generally assume that lower back pain is caused by a minor strain, sprain, pinched nerve (see page 38) or muscle knot that will go away of its own accord. These can be caused by an acute injury, such as lifting a wardrobe without due care and attention or bending over awkwardly, or chronic wear and tear from a slouchy posture, prolonged standing, sleeping on a saggy bed or long-distance driving. Being fat and unfit increases the risk because they increase the workload on an already-weak lower back.

There are other causes of lumbago which are far from trivial, can cause debilitating pain and discomfort and won't go away on their own. Slipped discs occur when a disc of cartilage between two vertebrae becomes displaced and presses painfully on a nerve. This is the main cause of sciatica, which is compression of the main nerve running from the lower back down to the feet. Then there are other, even worse but thankfully very rare causes, including deep-seated infections, arthritis and cancer. Persistent, debilitating and worsening lumbago needs to be checked out. But most cases will clear up. And then come back.

As well as lumbago, we humans are also plagued (though to a lesser extent) by middle and upper back pain. The causes are generally the same.

There are some obvious ways to reduce the risk of getting a painful back in the first place or it coming back. Stay active, lose weight, strengthen the core muscles, buy a decent mattress and maintain a good posture even when slumped at a desk or in front of the telly. Above all, take care when lifting heavy objects. Lifting things safely is not rocket science – lift with your legs not your back, get a firm grip, keep the load close to your body, plant feet firmly and apart, don't wear flip-flops. But huge numbers of people still end up putting their backs out by ignoring these simple rules.

If it is too late and lumbago is already stirring in your loins, there are a few things that can be done to relieve it: stretches and exercises like swimming and yoga, painkillers, and hot and cold compresses will all soothe and heal the injury. Or you could just give up on progress and go back to knuckle walking.

Trapped nerves

A trapped or pinched nerve is exactly what is sounds like. Sort of. For a variety of reasons, a nerve becomes compressed by surrounding tissue such as muscle or bone, causing shooting pains, numbness and pins and needles. One of the worst forms is sciatica (see page 36).

The main cause of trapped nerves is swelling around the nerve tunnel caused by an injury, wear and tear, or small outgrowths of bone called spurs which result from constant nagging friction on a bone. They can occur anywhere but are most common in the back, shoulder, arms, wrists and hands. Contrary to popular wisdom, a trapped nerve cannot be freed by opening up a joint, say by extending the spine. They are not literally 'trapped' between two bones. They generally clear up in a few weeks. As always, if they are bothering you and not getting better, be safe not sorry and see a doctor.

Gout

The UK Gout Society has a questionnaire on its website to check your own risk of getting gout. It consists of ten questions and if you answer yes to six or more, then it recommends a trip to the doctor. I took the questionnaire and, by the time I got to question seven, had clocked up six out of six. I am male, over forty, drink too much, have high blood pressure, a family history of gout, and am overweight (for the record, just a teeny bit).

But I don't have gout, yet. Of that I am very, very glad. Gout hurts like hell. A famous 1799 satirical drawing depicts gout as a fire-breathing imp sinking its fangs and claws into a red and swollen big toe. By all accounts this is genuinely what it feels like.

Gout is a form of arthritis, which is a general term for disease of the joints. The underlying cause is a build-up of uric acid in the blood which crystallises out as sodium urate in joints, bones and under the skin. In the joints these needle-shaped crystals can trigger a ferocious immune response that brings on excruciating pain, tenderness, heat, redness and swelling.

Attacks come on suddenly, often in the middle of the night. They can strike at any joint, though the most commonly afflicted are big toes, fingers, wrists, knees and elbows. The pain can be so bad that the lightest of touches, even from a bed sheet, is excruciating. People in the throes of a gout flare-up on a toe cannot put on socks, let alone shoes.

The creator of the fire-breathing imp was James Gillray, widely credited as the inventor of the political cartoon. He became notorious for satirising the high society of his time, including mad King George III; when Gillray himself developed gout in later life, there was no doubt a large amount of schadenfreude doing the rounds in the House of Hanover.

In Gillray's time, gout was believed to be a self-inflicted ailment of wealthy, middle-aged men who swilled claret and port and scoffed game pies and puddings with gluttonous abandon. That was deeply unfair; wealthy middle-aged women also got gout, including George III's corpulent predecessor Queen Anne. In the 1840s, doctors discovered that there was more to it than overindulgence, but the stereotype did not die. In his 1906 book *The Devil's Dictionary*, American satirist Ambrose Bierce defines it as 'a physician's name for the rheumatism of a rich patient'.

We now know that gout is principally a genetic disorder of metabolism which causes uric acid to build up faster than the kidneys can clear it out. Uric acid is produced by the metabolic breakdown of purines, which are a natural component of all foods. It is normally excreted in urine but due to various mutations some people cannot clear it fast enough, or make higher-than-usual amounts. The uric acid builds up in the blood and when it reaches a critical concentration crystallises out. The crystals are sometimes visible as small white lumps called tophi under the skin of the elbows, fingers and ears. These are a sign of chronic gout.

But gout cannot be entirely laid at the door of one's genes. Certain lifestyle choices can aggravate it in susceptible people, or even bring on an attack in people who are not. Some foods are especially rich in purines, including game meat, liver, kidneys, anchovies, mackerel, mussels and scallops. Beer is a prolific source, from the yeast used to brew it. Drinking too much alcohol in general is a risk factor. Eating a lot of sugar is another. Being overweight, inactive and unfit don't help. Nor does having high blood pressure. About 10 per cent of gout attacks appear to be caused purely by lifestyle factors; most others are lifestyle-related. Older men, who are more likely to have the risk factors, account for about 90 per cent of all cases. As with most stereotypes, it seems there is some truth in this one.

Severe gout can be treated with uric acid-lowering drugs but the first line of defence is painkillers, ice packs and drinking plenty of water. The pain usually subsides in a few agonised days. Doctors will also recommend lifestyle changes. You know the drill: lose weight, eat better, lay off the booze, exercise, stay hydrated. All of these will help to lower the uric acid concentration of the blood so that the crystals dissolve and the kidneys clear out the uric acid. Without them, another flare-up is only a matter of time.

Perhaps unsurprisingly, gout is on the increase in rich countries as people increasingly indulge in gouty lifestyles. In the UK, the prevalence rose by more than 50 per cent between 1997 and 2012. In the US about one in twenty-five people have gout.

Gout may feel like an archaic disease but it is probably more prevalent now than it was in its eighteenth-century heyday. In certain circles, gout is even being reclaimed as a status symbol. In 2018, the society magazine *Tatler* included it as a signifier of being upper class. It was tongue-in-cheek, but if and when I go down with gout I will take whatever comfort I can get.

Period pain and PMS

While writing this book I have often been able to draw on painful personal experience. But there is one common form of pain I can confidently say I have never endured and never will: period pain.

I have experienced somebody suffering from it, and it is no fun for either of us. It feels, apparently, like having your insides pulled out through your vagina. It starts in the lower abdomen on day one of the period and then spreads to the back. The pain is mostly constant, but occasionally peaks in short, sharp spasms. Every period brings pain, but some are worse than others.

That, at least, is my wife's experience of it. When I remind her that it will end soon, for ever, she shoots me a filthy look. It doesn't help that she is often really bloody humourless as well, but we will get to that.

Menstrual bleeding is the monthly-ish act of shedding the lining of the womb if a fertilised egg has not implanted in it (or sometimes if a genetically defective one has). After ovulation, the uterus prepares for a possible new occupant or three. The lining of the uterus – called the endometrium – proliferates, adding connective tissue and blood vessels to create a thick, spongy bed which will be a comfy place for a fertilised egg, or zygote, to bed down for a few months. The endometrium can more than quadruple in thickness from about 2 millimetres to 10 or more. But if a zygote does not arrive the uterus chucks it all away and starts again. The connective tissue dies and falls apart; small arteries in the endometrium rupture and start to flush the debris out. Over the course of a few days, the unwanted tissue and blood fall out of the vagina. The volume of blood lost ranges from about 30 to 90 millilitres.

The reason it hurts is because tissue is being torn from the uterus walls, which causes inflammation, and muscles in the uterus wall contract sharply to help flush the debris away. These are essentially the same as the contractions that occur in labour. Pains can carry on for up to seventy-two hours and, not coincidentally, are worse when the bleeding is heavy. Some women also get back or leg pains, bad breath or nausea.

Menstrual cramping – technically called dysmenor-rhea – is very common. About 85 per cent of women report enduring it; about half of these women say they get it every time they have a period. More than half of all women admit they need to take painkillers for their cramps and 40 per cent say that the pain is sometimes bad enough to keep them off school or work or interfere with their social life. Painkillers, hot water bottles, massage and exercise can ease the pain.

Why this has to happen is a biological conundrum. The vast majority of mammalian species have an oestrus cycle rather than a menstrual one. They do not jettison the lining of the womb, but simply re-absorb it. We can't ask them if it hurts, but it is a reasonable assumption that it does not.

The list of mammals that menstruate is a short and rather baffling one: great apes (including us), most old-world mon-keys, elephant shrews and two groups of bats, the free-tailed and leaf-nosed. What they have in common to favour men-struation is not clear.

If the pain and inconvenience of menstruation were not bad enough, around 80 per cent of women also experi-ence unpleasant physical and psychological changes in the days before their period. The symptoms of pre-menstrual syndrome (formerly and somewhat dismissively called pre-menstrual tension, or PMT) are many and varied and most women only have a few of them at any one time; be grateful for small mercies as they include mood swings, irritability, anxiety, tearfulness, insomnia, fatigue, tender breasts, headaches, abdominal pain, water retention, loss of appetite, changes in libido, zits and greasy hair. Like period pain, they often vary from month to month. They usually go away once the bleeding starts. Some women report having them for up to two weeks before they come on, giving them a glorious week free of menstrual troubles per month.

The cause of PMS is not known, but is usually put rather vaguely down to 'hormones'. Or, in some circles, to women's fertile imaginations. PMT was once dismissed as yet another manifestation of female irrationality and tendency towards hysteria. There is still some controversy around it, with some critics arguing that it is a social construct rather than a medical phenomenon. In this minority view women are socially conditioned to expect pre-menstrual symptoms and so they will them into existence.

As somebody who lives with a woman who experiences varying levels of pre-menstrual syndrome, I think this is total and utter garbage. As with her period pains, I sometimes point out to my wife that, as a woman in her early fifties, she can look forward to a PMS-free near future. But she is usually in NO MOOD to hear this.

Toothache

My maternal grandmother always used to warn me and my sister about the dangers of eating sweets. 'You don't want to end up like me!' she would say, clacking her dentures. As a child she had had all of her teeth – every single one of them – removed, and wore dentures for more than fifty years. She had a lovely smile. But her advice on sweets went unheeded. I still have most of my teeth.

I can't help wondering if my grandma wasn't a victim of one of the early twentieth century's oddest medical fads: the total removal of teeth, often from young women, often as an eighteenth or twenty-first birthday present, which were then replaced with perfectly white and straight dentures. Admittedly, snaggly British teeth have never had much of a reputation for aesthetic beauty, and even back then a Hollywood smile was a desirable thing. But it was also done to spare the unfortunate girl a lifetime of toothache, dentistry and pulled teeth, and the hefty bills that would surely follow. Might as well get it all over and done with, eh?

Dentistry is still a costly business, but prophylactic tooth pulling is now only practised where there is a serious medical need. Those of us with teeth (and a sweet tooth) do have to suffer occasional bouts of toothache. But that is surely better than lifelong toothlessness.

Teeth are an undeniably useful but annoyingly error-prone piece of anatomy. The hard outer part – the enamel – is neither as hard nor as thick as we'd like it to be, and the teeth and spaces between them offer plenty of lodging for morsels of food and hence colonies of bacteria to thrive. These cause bad breath and gum disease (see page 174), and also rot our teeth.

Tooth decay is not actual rot, as in the microbial putrefaction of dead organic matter. It is caused by acids excreted by a class of mouth-dwelling bacteria called cariogens, because they cause dental caries. They eat sugar and poo out lactic acid which, over time, erodes the enamel and eventually breaches it. Enamel is the hardest tissue in the human body – it is 96 per cent hydroxyapatite, a white crystalline form of calcium phosphate – but even this cannot withstand years of acid attack. Once the enamel is breached the game is essentially up. The acid then makes a start on the dentin, the layer under the enamel which is also mostly hydroxyapatite, though softer because it contains more water and organic compounds. Acid attack on the outer layers of the tooth does not hurt, but once they are breached, the internal pulp, which is living tissue with sensitive nerve endings, is exposed. Ouch. A filling beckons.

Hot and cold food or drinks can jolt the pain, for obvious reasons. So can sugar, for less obvious ones. It can directly irritate the nerve endings in the exposed pulp and also up the production of lactic acid.

Other acids are cariogenic too, especially the phosphoric acid that is often added to fizzy drinks to add tang. Some people worry that sparkling water erodes tooth enamel, but it does not. It is slightly acidic because the bubbles are carbon dioxide, which dissolves in water to form carbonic acid. But the acid is too weak to dissolve enamel.

Dental caries are very common. Figures collected by the US National Health and Nutrition Examination Survey found that adults aged twenty to sixty-nine had, on average, seven fillings and two-and-a-half missing teeth.[12] A quarter had untreated tooth decay.

Not getting treatment is a bad idea, especially if the motivation is to avoid the dentist. Once a tooth has a hole in it, treatment is the only way back. If decay goes untreated it can lead to an infection of the pulp which can spread into the roots of the tooth and cause an abscess – a sac of pus that needs to be drained, cleaned and disinfected in a dreaded procedure called a root canal. Avoiding the simple and usually painless procedure of getting a filling can lead to much worse.

When I were a lad, fillings were invariably made of amalgam, or 'silver fillings'. Amalgam is a really good filling material as it is soft when fresh but hardens quickly and can endure decades of chewing. But it also causes much gnashing of teeth. It is an alloy of silver, tin, zinc and, gulp, mercury. That sounds like a dangerous mixture to carry around in your mouth for decades: isn't mercury a deadly poison? It is, but its elemental metallic form is largely benign. It is also very stable and just sits there in the filling doing nothing, especially in the presence of zinc, which is more easily oxidised and so stops the mercury atoms from being converted into dangerous mercury ions. This is the same principle as galvanisation. If you have amalgam fillings, your teeth are galvanised.

There is some evidence of mild heavy metal toxicity from amalgam fillings, though also that having them removed can be a risk because it releases mercury that would otherwise do no harm. Current advice is to leave them in place unless they are damaged or there is decay underneath them. Nonetheless, new amalgam fillings are gradually being phased out in favour of polymer resins, which have the advantage of being white but are less durable.

If you want to avoid having painful teeth, a gob full of mercury or a root canal, dental hygiene is the answer. If you live in an area without fluoridated water, choose fluoridated toothpaste as fluorine ions are chemically incorporated into the tooth enamel and strengthen it. There is even some evidence that fluorine can help repair early-stage tooth decay.

Fluoridation of the water supply makes some people nervous, usually libertarians who see it as an infringement of their freedom to have tooth decay. But the US Centers for Disease Control and Prevention says that water fluoridation is proven to prevent caries and is 'one of ten great public health achievements of the twentieth century'. For some reason, the mass removal of teeth does not make the list.

No amount of dental hygiene can protect from another common cause of toothache: the dreaded 'third molars', commonly called wisdom teeth. These usually erupt in people's late teens or early twenties (which is an interesting definition of 'wisdom'). Some lucky people never get them; they are there in the jaw but for some reason do not erupt.

Wisdom teeth are an evolutionary throwback to a time when our ancestors derived a lot of their calories from fibrous foods that required vigorous and lengthy mastication. By their late teens, their other eight molars were probably shot and backups were required.

We no longer really need them and, annoyingly, our jaws have shrunk somewhat over the past 50,000 years or so, so there often isn't room to accommodate them. They can push against the incumbent molars and cause tooth and jaw pain. The answer: whip them out, though dental authorities now advise against routine removal if they are not causing bother. Now that really is wisdom. Belatedly.

2

The Skin You're in

2

The Skin You're In

Here's a classic quiz question: what is the largest organ in the human body? The liver? The lungs? No – it is, of course, the skin. We don't often think of skin as an organ, but it is, and a vital one at that. It's the boundary between you and the rest of the world and, like a nightclub bouncer, strictly controls who and what can come in. It's hugely varied, from the delicate patina of our faces to the rhinoceros-like hide on the bottom of our feet. And it's big: the external surface area of an average human is about 2 square metres, and weighs about 4 kilograms.

Being so big, a lot can go wrong. And being so visible, unpleasantly so. Some of the most embarrassing and distressing minor ailments are found on the skin: acne, scabies, dandruff, rashes. We'll encounter all of them in this section, and more besides. But let's start with the minor ailment that inspired me to write this book: the common-or-garden but also cunning and fascinating disease called 'squamous cell papilloma'. Or, in common parlance, warts.

Warts

In 1657, six years after finally winning the English Civil Wars, Oliver Cromwell decided it was time to inject some pomp and ceremony into his otherwise dour and puritanical reign. The Lord Protector of the erstwhile Republic of England, Scotland and Ireland was not renowned as a barrel of laughs; he was a strict disciplinarian who despised all forms of flummery. But in a bout of narcissism he commissioned the Dutch-born artist Peter Lely to paint him an official portrait. Lely was probably as relieved as he was surprised. Just four years earlier Cromwell had usurped and beheaded his former master, King Charles I, and purged the court of his followers.

Royal portrait artists were expected to flatter their subjects but Cromwell clearly decided his ego could only take so much massaging. 'Mr Lely,' he is reported to have said, 'I desire you would use all your skill to paint my picture truly like me, and not flatter me at all; but remark all these roughnesses, pimples, warts, and everything as you see me; otherwise I will never pay a farthing for it.' This (possibly apocryphal) quote was later shortened to 'paint me, warts and all.'

Whether Cromwell actually had warts is not known. His portrait does not show them – maybe Lely thought flattery was a good idea after all – and his death mask reveals only what looks like a large mole above the right eyebrow, which may have been what he was asking Lely to paint.

But it would be no surprise if he did have warts. They are among the most common of minor ailments. Almost everyone gets one at some point in their life and at any one time about 10 per cent of us is sporting one somewhere. They are hard to get rid of, though generally clear up by themselves, eventually. They are usually painless – though the ones on the soles of the feet, commonly known as verrucas (derived from a Latin word meaning 'little hill'), can really hurt. But they are annoying and ugly, especially for the unfortunate people who get them on their face.

As Cromwell clearly knew, warts are generally regarded as an unflattering affliction: warty toads and warthogs are not noted for their physical beauty. Handling or killing toads was a common folk theory for the origin of warts, as was washing hands in water in which eggs have been boiled and, of course, masturbation. In the late Middle Ages, warts were regarded as a devil's mark and women who had them on their faces were often accused of witchcraft.

That was, of course, deeply unfair. Warts can and do affect anyone. Technically they are classed as a type of tumour, which sounds serious but simply means 'swelling' in Latin.

Warts are actually a viral infection of a deep layer of your skin; their viral origin was discovered in 1907 when an Italian doctor called Giuseppe Ciuffo gave himself warts by inoculating himself with an 'extract of wart' that had been passed through a filter fine enough to exclude bacteria and fungi.

The culprit is the human papillomavirus (HPV), of which there are around 130 varieties. Most don't cause warts. In fact, most don't seem to cause anything. A few of them cause cancer, which is why schoolchildren are often vaccinated against them aged twelve or thirteen. But the ones causing common-or-garden warts – not the genital variety, which are emphatically not a minor ailment because they can progress to cancer and hence require medical attention – are not carcinogenic.

HPV comes in two types: 'low risk' (wart causing) or 'high risk' (cancer causing). I'm going to limit myself in this book to the low-risk ones here.

HPV is a small virus. At roughly 55 nanometres across, it's about a thousandth of the width of a human hair. It consists of a loop of double-stranded DNA containing eight genes encased in protein armour called a capsid. Under an electron microscope it looks like a regular polyhedron with seventy-two faces.

People often imagine that viruses are evil little geniuses with malign intent towards us, but that is unfair and scientifically inaccurate. Most biologists don't even class viruses as living things because they are so utterly dependent on their host's metabolism to feed themselves and reproduce. They have no purpose or goal. They are merely molecular parasites that have stumbled across loopholes in our biology to mindlessly reproduce themselves. Such is non-life.

HPV is easy to catch. People with warts shed the virus constantly, onto anything they touch or walk on with bare feet. You can pick a wart virus up by direct skin contact or by touching something contaminated, such as a towel or the floor of a locker room. However, mere contact is not enough. The virus has to get lucky and land on some skin with a minor cut that provides access to its target, a layer of tissue called the basal epithelium. This is the deepest of five layers of skin cells; it is a factory for cells called corneocytes that go on to form the outer layer of the skin. These cells are essentially dead.

The virus's need to penetrate deep into the skin is why damp and rough areas such as the edges of swimming pools are especially conducive to transmission, as wet skin on the soles of the feet is softened and more easily grazed. This is why swimming pools herd people through a disinfectant foot bath and ask those with verrucas to wear special plastic socks. But they are fighting a losing battle. British Swimming, the sport's national governing body, now accepts that 'to place resources into eradicating verrucas is a waste of time'.

Soon after infecting a cell, the viral genome commandeers its DNA-replicating machinery and produces around 100 copies of itself, then slips into sleeper mode as the skin cell proliferates and its daughters begin their three-week journey to the outermost layer. But even with the virus lying dormant, each daughter cell is born with 100 or so viral genomes inside it, producing thousands of sleeper cells primed with viral DNA.

The next stage occurs in a layer of the skin closer to the surface called the 'differentiating compartment', where cells normally stop dividing and begin to differentiate into cells that will head to the surface for their brief day in the sun. At this point – the cue is unclear – the sleeper cells spring into action and replicate their viral DNA like crazy, producing thousands of copies of the viral genome and the protein building blocks that are required to build new viruses.

The resulting cells are not typical outer skin cells, but zombies that are entirely dedicated to producing new virus particles. When they finally reach the skin's surface they are little more than dead sacks of virus, which gives the wart its rough, cauliflower-like appearance and texture. Warts also often have small black dots inside them; these are tiny blood clots from minor bleeds caused by the rampaging growth of the zombified cells.

The size of the wart depends on how many basal cells are infected. The largest can be several centimetres across.

Roughly speaking there are three categories of regular wart: the common wart (verruca vulgaris), the plantar wart (verruca plantaris) and the flat wart (verruca plana). Common warts usually occur on the hands, plantar warts on the soles of the feet (an area that anatomists call the 'plantar') and flat warts on the face and legs, sometimes in clusters of up to 100. They usually don't cause any discomfort, though plantar warts on load-bearing areas of the sole can be painful because the pressure of walking pushes them against the underlying layers of skin.

The most common type are plantar warts, which account for almost half of cases. A further third are common warts, usually on the hands, and about 15 per cent of cases are flat warts, mostly facial.

As you might expect, the three types are often caused by different subtypes of the virus, though not always. Subtype 3, for example, can cause common and flat warts, while Types 1 and 2 can cause common and plantar warts. Exactly why the same virus can produce such different growths is not known.

Sometimes, for reasons also unknown, an even stranger structure can appear. Some warts grow a cluster of long, thin filaments not unlike the tentacles of a sea anemone or sausage meat being extruded from a tiny mincer. These curious-looking filiform warts usually appear on the face, most frequently around the eyes and lips. They look a bit like skin tags (see page 59) but are not the same thing.

Another less common type is the butcher's wart, which – as its name suggests – usually affects the hands of people who frequently handle raw meat. Butcher's warts appear to be associated with HPV7, though why there is a connection between it and meat isn't known. Other mammals have their own wart-causing papilloma viruses – they have been recorded in dogs, cows, sheep, deer, rabbits and pigs (which suggests that warthogs have warts too) – but they appear to be highly species-specific.

There may be some bizarre connection between the butcher's wart and the many common folk remedies for warts that are based on raw meat. One version, advocated by my wife's late grandmother, is to steal some meat from somebody else's larder, rub it on the wart and bury the meat in your garden. This practice is inadvisable for both legal and medical reasons; it's far more likely to cause warts than cure them.

Other folk cures for warts are equally bizarre and ineffective, usually involving disgusting or smelly things – dog dirt, pig blood, fish heads. One is to rub the wart with a large black slug and then impale the unfortunate slug on a thorn. Swedish peasants apparently used a species of bush cricket to nibble at their warts; both its Latin (*Decticus verrucivorus*) and common name (*Warzenbeisser*) mean 'wart eater'.

The desperate and sometimes extreme nature of these folk remedies are probably testament to the persistence and tenacity of warts. Once in, the viruses are hard to dislodge. Infected cells carry on churning out infected daughter cells which continue to feed the wart. Left untreated, warts can persist for months or even years.

Their persistence is because the virus is extremely cunning, making itself almost invisible to the immune system. Unlike most viruses, HPV does not need to explode out of its host cell like soldiers disgorging from a Trojan horse to complete its life cycle. That occurs automatically when the skin cell reaches the surface.

The virus is further advantaged because the outer skin cells are destined for death and ejection anyway, so the immune system does not keep them under tight surveillance. Normal cues that a cell is infected – such as viral proteins being expressed on the cell surface – are absent. In addition, the virus has evolved a sneaky way of spiking the infected cells' anti-viral guns, the interferon genes. These produce proteins called interferons which are the body's natural antivirals and also send out an SOS to the immune system. Without them, another of the immune system's alarm bells fails to ring.

But eventually the virus slips up and exposes itself to the immune system. What follows is swift and ruthless: white blood cells known as killer-T cells rush to the base of the wart and unleash chemical warfare on the infected cells, killing them. Over the next few weeks, the wart, now deprived of new recruits, shrivels and eventually falls off. Around two-thirds of warts are wiped out this way within two years, and 80 per cent within four.

Many people don't wait that long, choosing to unleash their own form of chemical warfare. Pharmacy shelves are groaning with expensive cures, which, as British Swimming points out, is 'principally because none of them work satisfactorily'.

The first line of treatment is usually salicylic acid, an organic acid related to aspirin which dissolves the outer layer of skin and is also used to treat acne, ringworm, dandruff, calluses and corns. The idea is that the acid gradually eats its way down to the basal layer and kills off the source of the problem.

Alternative treatments include other acids, antiviral drugs or even liquid nitrogen to freeze the wart to death. Some very persistent warts require stronger medicine such as lasers, pulses of electricity or surgery. But as one recent review paper warns: 'Even though there are many treatments for warts, none is very effective, and recurrences are common with each of them.' Unless your wart is painful or unsightly, you are better off letting nature take its course.[13]

Another reason for doing so is that once the wart is destroyed, the immune system remembers the virus and confers lifelong immunity to it. This is why warts are more common among children and adolescents than adults. It is also why an outbreak of warts in an adult can be a warning sign of immune dysfunction.

While you wait for your wart to shrivel and die, remember that it is constantly shedding potential baby warts. Don't pick at warts or hack at them with an emery board or razor blade as you may spread them to other parts of your skin, and don't bite your fingernails as you may create a new entry point for the virus to exploit.

And remember, warts are a human universal. So you might as well reconcile yourself to sharing your skin with one for a while. Whatever the adverts say, there's probably not much point trying to bazooka your verruca. Instead, take a lesson from the famously stoic Oliver Cromwell and just accept the skin you're in, warts and all.

Skin tags

Sometimes skin does not need to be invaded by a virus to grow an unsightly little blob. Skin tags look a bit like warts but are actually just small, squishy and wrinkly blobs of skin. They are not flush to the surface like moles but dangle pendulously from a stalk, not unlike a miniature testicle – fortunately *very* miniature, as they usually grow no bigger than 5 millimetres across. Tags mostly sprout on the neck, armpits, groin and under the breasts but can grow anywhere. They are totally harmless, neither cancerous nor contagious, though they can chafe on zips and jewellery and are a real pain when shaving.

What triggers skin tags is not known, though they are more common in people who are obese, diabetic or pregnant. The fact that they are common in skin folds has led to the suggestion that they are some kind of response to repeated friction. There is also a genetic component as they run in families.

Once a skin tag has grown, it is just as much a part of your body as, say, your leg. Very occasionally they fall off, possibly as a result of the stalk becoming twisted and the blood supply being cut off. But mostly they just sit there. Do not attempt to remove them yourself unless you are a fan of copious bleeding. Removal by surgery, ligation or freezing is possible but they often just grow back.

Zits, blackheads and acne

Zits seem like one of nature's cruel jokes. Puberty arrives, childish things are put away, thoughts turn to more adult pastimes. Then, bang, your face turns into a pizza.

Teenage spots and acne, almost universally known as zits, are an unfortunate fact of life. Very few of us never get one, and about 95 per cent of people aged eleven to thirty experience at least one outbreak severe enough to qualify as mild acne. (There is actually no formal threshold at which the odd spot becomes acne, but a cluster of fifteen or more would usually be diagnosed as a mild case.)

Zits may seem like a skin condition but are actually a disorder of an organ called the pilosebaceous unit, commonly called the hair follicle. Think of them as a bad hair-follicle day. Each unit consists of a narrow pit in the skin with a hair root at the bottom, plus one or more sebaceous glands. These secrete a yellowish waxy substance called sebum into the follicle and thence out onto the surface of the skin. Sebum is widely believed to lubricate the hair and skin but actually has no known function.[14] Young children do not produce sebum; neither does the skin on the palms of the hands and soles of the feet. All function perfectly well without it.

Sometimes the follicle becomes clogged up with sebum, dead skin and other detritus, and that is how zits start. Clogged follicles are technically called comedones, and come in two forms: whiteheads and blackheads. If these are not unclogged they can progress to worse and worse types of zit – papules, pustules, nodules and cysts. An outbreak of any of these on the face, back or chest is called acne vulgaris, or common acne.

These areas are prone to acne because of their high density of hair follicles. You may not think of them as especially hirsute, but they are. Follicle for follicle, humans are as hairy as chimps. We typically have about 5 million hairs on our head and body, about the same as any other primate. They are all over the skin except for the palms of the hands and the soles of the feet. The reason we appear largely hairless is that most of our hairs are short, wispy and invisible to the naked eye (this is also true of men who lose their head hair; they are not actually bald but just very delicately hirsute).

Unfortunately, that illusion of hairlessness also exposes our diseased follicles to the outside world for all to see.

The reason comedones form two different types of zit has to do with the location of the blockage. If the debris is confined within the pore and causes the skin to bulge outwards, it is a whitehead.

If some of the debris is oozing out of the follicle it can react with oxygen in the air, turning it a dark colour and producing a blackhead. Blackheads are also black because the skin inside the hair follicle can contain the dark brown pigment melanin.

Comedones are the least worst type of zit as they do not – yet – involve inflammation, so are painless and don't have that angry red pizza colour. Blackheads are the easiest to get rid of because the comedo is already open to the outside world so the blockage can be flushed out; whiteheads are trickier because the blockage is trapped under the skin. Both can be treated quite effectively with facial cleansers containing the mild acid salicylic acid (also used to treat warts) or the antiseptic benzoyl peroxide. These are readily available in over-the-counter remedies. Tea tree oil, extracted from a shrub native to Australia, is commonly used for the same purpose but the evidence for its effectiveness is limited.

Another common method of expelling debris is to 'open the pores' using steam, hot water or hot towels. This may help to keep the skin clean but the follicles themselves do not open or close. Some people naturally have larger follicles than others and large follicles can be prone to blockages, but their size is not something we can control.

Blackheads and whiteheads can also be squeezed to expel the debris, but dermatologists advise against this because it can cause scarring and, in the case of whiteheads, backfire, forcing the debris deeper into the follicle and making it more likely that it will progress to the next level.

Before we get on to that, however, it is worth mentioning 'fool's blackheads', or sebaceous filaments. These are thin strands of dried sebum and the tough structural protein keratin that protrude out of unblocked follicles, especially the large ones on the nose. They are dark in colour like blackheads and are often mistaken for them, but are not a blockage – they are just sebum doing what sebum does, which is to ooze out of follicles like slow-moving treacle. Avoid the temptation to squeeze them out as you may turn a perfectly healthy follicle into an inflamed one, a.k.a. a zit.

Anyway, time to go to that next level. If comedones become infected by bacteria that normally live harmlessly on the skin, particularly the cutely named sebum eater *Cutibacterium acnes*, they can become inflamed, painful and red. This happens more easily with whiteheads than blackheads because they are buried under the surface and there is no way to flush out the bacteria; for this reason whiteheads have been described as the 'time bombs' of acne. The infection causes the whitehead to become inflamed and sore; at this point it has become a papule. If pus – the remains of dead white blood cells that perished fighting the infection – accumulates and forms a visible white or yellowish head, it has been further upgraded to a pustule, the classic zit that has come to a head. Most pustules eventually burst of their own accord (or are deliberately squeezed, though again the squeezing of zits is frowned upon by dermatologists) and the follicle then heals. But sometimes the infection burrows deeper into the follicle, rupturing and destroying it completely and forming large pus-filled lesions called nodules which can amalgamate with neighbouring ones to form cysts. These deep and long-lasting superzits are painful, unsightly and often lead to scarring. They require medical attention.

Nodules and cysts can sometimes appear in isolation, without a case of acne, in which case they are known as boils and carbuncles. They, too, are caused by an infection of the hair follicle and require similar treatment.

Spots are painful because the associated inflammation stretches the skin and triggers pain receptors to fire. This is especially problematic where the skin is taut, thin and sensitive, such as on the edge of the nostril. A friend of mine once broke his arm snowboarding. When his wife asked him how much it hurt, he said, 'A lot, but not as much as one of those zits inside your nose.'

The worst spot I've ever had was a nasal one, but it was not caused by a blocked follicle. It erupted on the side of my nose about a week before we were due to attend a friend's wedding. I thought it would go away in time but it just grew and grew. Every day was a personal red nose day; by the time the big day came round I looked like a zitty Pinocchio. My entire nose was swollen, red and painful; it was not the most relaxed social occasion I've ever experienced. About a week later, the spot finally came to a head and I squeezed it. There was a lot of pus and some instant pain relief but I also noticed a small black dot in the middle of the wreckage. I got some tweezers and pulled at it, whereupon it started to unravel like a loose thread on a jumper. I kept on pulling; it kept on unravelling. Eventually the whole thing came loose, along with yet more pus. It was a hair about 5 centimetres long that had evidently grown inwards from my nostril, burrowing through the flesh of my nose and out the other side.

My Pinocchio nose turned out to be caused by a pseudo-folliculitis barbae, or ingrown hair. These occur when a growing hair curls round in itself and burrows back into the follicle. They are especially common in people with curly hair – tick – who shave or trim their unwanted body or facial hair – tick. Men with tightly curled facial hair who shave closely are especially prone. Ingrowing hairs are harmless but painful and unsightly, and I can tell you from personal experience that getting shot of one is extremely satisfying. If you want to experience the relief vicariously, there are a number of YouTube channels dedicated to footage of ingrowing hairs being removed. They are worryingly compelling.

In fact, footage of people having their zits, boils and other pus-filled skin lesions popped and drained is something of a niche internet sensation. One YouTuber, dermatologist Dr Sandra Lee, even landed her own TV show, *Dr Pimple Popper*, which ran to four seasons on cable channel TLC. It later spawned a spinoff called, brilliantly, *This Is Zit*.

Some people are more prone to acne than others, largely due to genetic factors that endow them with larger hair follicles and more productive sebaceous glands, a combination commonly known as oily skin. The glands are also sensitive to surges of sex hormones such as testosterone and oestrogen, which also cause mood disorders and are why pubescent teens are often spotty little oiks.

Like many an unsightly skin disorder, acne is often blamed on the victims. This is grossly unfair. Some of the things that do not cause acne are greasy food, dirty skin, snogging other people with acne and masturbation. But keep hair clean and don't let if flop over your forehead, as this can make zits worse. Greasy hair is also caused by overactive sebaceous glands so people who are already battling an oily complexion have to be extra careful about this.

There is also no evidence that exposure to sunlight can help clear it up. Frequent face-washing can also make it worse because it irritates the skin. If over-the-counter remedies don't help, your doctor will be able to prescribe medication such as antibiotics. They are not especially effective, but time is a great healer. Most people's acne peaks in the late teens and has cleared up by the time they are thirty, just in time for your first wrinkles. Mother Nature can be a cruel mistress.

Rashes

Technically speaking, acne is a type of rash, not that that is an especially useful medical fact. The word 'rash' can apply to so many different things with so many different causes that it is practically useless. By definition it is simply a change in the colour, texture or appearance of the skin. That could mean almost anything, including the time my younger son drew blotches all over his face with red felt pen. An *indelible* red felt pen. He was angling for a day off school due to a nasty bout of lazyitis. It didn't wash, in either sense of the word.

Rashes can be caused by a long list of minor and major ailments including allergies, irritants, infectious diseases, parasites such as scabies (see page 270), skin diseases, bites and stings from insects and other invertebrates, too much sun or heat, too much cold, or too much cold followed by too much heat.

Infectious diseases such as viruses and bacteria cause rashes in two ways: either the pathogen deliberately creates a rash to further its own agenda, such as with chickenpox (see page 242). Or the immune response to it creates inflammation of the skin above where the virus is actively replicating.

The NHS lists seventeen causes of rashes in babies and young children, most of them entirely harmless, but a few rashes call for urgent medical attention. This is not a book about serious diseases but I feel duty bound to mention the most serious of these, meningitis, which is a potentially fatal infection of the membranes surrounding the brain. A rash on the body that does not fade when a glass is pressed against it is a classic symptom of meningitis. The other warning signs of meningitis are: stiff neck, aversion to bright light, uncontrollable shaking, uncontrollable fever, confusion and unusually cold hands and/or feet. Any of these on their own is a good reason to seek help; two or more add up to an emergency. Do not delay.

Most rashes, both in childhood and adulthood, are nowhere near as serious. I'll deal with most of them piece-meal in the appropriate chapters. But one that does not merit any further attention is an outbreak of red felt pen. I can tell you from experience that that is harmless and clears up on its own, but only after a few weeks. Of embarrassment.

Dermatitis (eczema)

One of the common causes of rashes is inflammation, which is a generalised immune response to a potential threat. When this occurs to the skin – also called the dermis – the result is dermatitis.

Commonly called eczema, from the Greek *ékzema*, 'to boil over', dermatitis is characterised by itchiness, dryness and/or a rash. The rash is usually red on pale skin; rashes on brown or black skin are often darker brown, purple or grey.

Dermatitis is classified into three major categories: contact, atopic and static. As the name suggests, contact dermatitis is caused by the skin coming into contact with something that doesn't agree with it. That might be an allergen, chemical irritant or a razor-sharp piece of metal (see page 316). Some things that are explicitly designed to be brought into contact with the skin, such as soap, shampoo, cosmetics and moisturiser, can trigger dermatitis in some people. Even prolonged exposure to water can bring it on, though actual water allergy is extraordinarily rare.[15]

One type of contact dermatitis I haven't had for about half a century, though can't be entirely confident of never getting again, is irritant napkin dermatitis or nappy rash (diaper rash to speakers of American English). This is usually caused by – there is no delicate way to put this – prolonged contact with urine or faeces. Or both. The wetness causes friction between the nappy and the skin, causing mild abrasions of the buttocks. The result is an angry-looking circular rash, often with pimples, blisters or flaky skin.

The combination of urine and faeces is especially potent as digestive enzymes in the faeces break down uric acid in the urine to release the alkaline chemical ammonia, which both corrodes the skin directly and neutralises its usual slight acidity, making it easier to breach. This is exacerbated by the fact that young children's backsides really are as soft as the proverbial baby's bum. The skin is not fully developed as a defensive barrier, so breaks down quite easily under friction and chemical attack.

About a third of babies and toddlers get nappy rash at some point during their nappy-wearing months. They can also get another sub-category of dermatitis, called seborrheic dermatitis (more commonly called dandruff, or cradle cap in babies; see page 72) in that area. Arse dandruff.

Nappy rash usually doesn't cause babies too much bother, but can become sore, especially if the rash becomes infected with bacteria or fungi. Prevention and cure are no-brainers. Apply nappy-rash creams, change nappies often, don't let kids sit around in their own poo and wee and leave them out of nappies for a while whenever possible. It might get messy, but bear in mind that you may be in a position to extract payback one day. I won't dwell on that but three words will suffice: incontinence-associated dermatitis.

Another type of dermatitis that used to bother me but cleared up years ago is atopic dermatitis. This is the classic eczema that breaks out for no apparent reason behind knees and ears and elbows, often in children, and persists stubbornly for months or years. I mostly had it behind my ears – it used to create crusty scabs that I found weirdly pleasurable to pick off, though other people were less enamoured – and also blepharitis, which is eczema of the eyelids (see page 104).

The exact cause of atopic dermatitis (which comes from the word 'atopy', meaning the tendency to have an exaggerated immune response to harmless stimuli) is unknown, but it runs in families and clearly has a strong genetic component. If one identical twin has it, the other has an 85 per cent chance of having it too. It is also linked to immune system dysfunction, as it tends to co-occur with asthma and allergies. It seems to be exacerbated by stress, but stress has been ruled out as a direct cause. I still get a bit of it at stressy times, such as when trying to hit a book deadline. But don't worry, I am leaving my ear scabs alone.

Contact and atopic dermatitis are dealt with in the same way, using moisturisers to help the skin heal and steroid creams to damp down the inflammation.

The third type of dermatitis, stasis, is less common and rather nasty. It is caused by blood pooling in veins and tissues in the legs under the influence of gravity – hence an alternative name, gravitational eczema – perhaps due to progressive weakening and dysfunction of the blood vessel walls or the valves that stop the blood from flowing in the wrong direction. This is also the cause of varicose veins (see page 119), and the two conditions are associated – hence another alternative name, varicose dermatitis. As well as the itchiness and rash it can progress to ulceration. It is quite serious and requires medical attention.

A word about '-itis'

Given how common and varied dermatitis is, this seems a good time to tackle the '-itis' issue. The word '-itis' is a catch-all suffix to indicate that some part of the body is inflamed, but is woefully misused. Though admittedly often in the service of humour, so crimes against it can be forgiven.

It is ultimately derived from the Ancient Greek word *ítis*, meaning 'pertaining to', which was often used in conjunction with the word for disease, *nosos*. So disease of the joints was called 'arthritis nosos' – in other words, a disease pertaining to the body's articulations. Nosos was eventually dropped, leaving '-itis' standing alone.

Arthritis was one of the first '-itis' words to find its way into English; it is known from the sixteenth century. But it caught on big time and there are now hundreds of official 'itises'.

Think of the name of a body part, usually in Latin or Greek, and chances are you can stick 'itis' onto the end of it to create an inflammatory ailment. There are dozens mentioned in this book and many more that are not because they are far from minor (think encephalitis, hepatitis, appendicitis).

'Itis' has also become a catch-all suffix for humorous fictional diseases, as in lazyitis, coined by the Happy Mondays in their typically tuneless song of the same name. A pedant would point out that lazyitis is not a correct usage, as the lazy is not a body part that can become inflamed. They might also point out that there is a fictional condition called Mondayitis. I am not that guy.

Flaky skin and dandruff

It's a good job babies are not self-conscious, because if they were, their terrible dandruff would be a cause of mortal embarrassment. It's not helped by being bald, but having a scalp covered in greasy yellow or brown crusts is not a good look, especially when you're supposed to be working on your cuteness. Sometimes it also encrusts the eyebrows and what is delicately called the 'nappy area'. We give it a cute name, cradle cap, but let's call a spade a spade – it is actually really bad dandruff, or, to use proper medical terminology, seborrheic dermatitis.

As the name suggests, this is a skin inflammation that affects areas with a high density of sebaceous glands. That includes the scalp, sides of the nose, eyebrows, ears and chest. Its cause is unknown – it may be a form of atopic dermatitis, meaning it is caused by an irregular immune response, or it may be due to an infection of the hair follicles, possibly by a sebum-eating yeast called *Malassezia*.

Seborrheic dermatitis is not the only cause of dandruff. Other forms of dermatitis (see page 68) can also afflict the scalp and cause it to become dry and flaky. But it is one of the most common and stubborn. It has nothing to do with poor cleanliness, which is still commonly though unfairly blamed for dandruff. If it were true, half of us would need to look in the mirror – and brush away some small white pieces of dead skin that have flaked off the scalp and fallen like snow onto the shoulders.

Flaky or scaly skin – known medically as pityriasis, derived from the Greek word for bran – can affect almost any part of the body. Another common cause is psoriasis, which is characterised by the formation of flaky red patches coated in silvery scales on the elbows, knees, lower back and scalp. It is caused by too-rapid turnover of skin cells, which normally takes three to four weeks but is reduced to a few days with psoriasis. The cause is unknown. Psoriasis of the scalp is another leading cause of dandruff.

In the case of cradle cap, the dandruff does not flake and fall off but becomes stuck in excess sebum and forms greasy crusts. They are easily removed – though often take a clump of baby hair with them – and the condition usually clears up in a few months.

Flaky skin disorders are almost always nothing to worry about and can be controlled by creams and shampoos, but are often a cause of embarrassment. We should all channel our inner babies and just style it out.

Itching

The Florentine poet Dante knew a thing or two about torture. In *Inferno* – the first part of his epic poem *Divine Comedy* – he describes the many agonies that sinners will be subjected to in the nine circles of hell. Gluttons are forced to wallow in freezing slush; heretics are trapped in flaming tombs; suicides are gnawed at by harpies. The worst fate of all is in the innermost circle, where traitors of various kinds are immersed in a freezing lake. But the second-worst form of torture is meted out to falsifiers such as frauds, forgers and impostors. Among other things, they are tormented by 'the great rage of itching' that even scratching off their skin cannot relieve.

Dante was a man of his time and was probably influenced by a form of torment that was widely practised by medieval sinners even before they were dispatched to hell. Christian penitents often wore a hair shirt – also called a cilice – to produce a constant, maddening itch. They were made of coarse sackcloth or animal hair, though some enthusiasts added twigs for extra irritation.

Hair shirts have fallen out of fashion but it is not hard to imagine how insanely annoying wearing one must have been; who hasn't railed at an itchy label in a T-shirt or pair of undies, or itched all day after a haircut?

But even without an obvious source, most of us are tormented by itches from time to time. Itching is the most common complaint encountered by dermatologists. Despite this, it remains largely mysterious. Though the cause is sometimes obvious and treatable, about a third of itches have no known origin.

In medical circles, itching is called pruritus, which is derived from the Latin word for 'itchy burning'. (The word 'prurient', which means taking an excessive interest in sex, has the same root.) The common name comes from the Old English word ʒiccan, 'to itch' (ʒ is the archaic letter yogh, pronounced 'y'; the double-c is pronounced 'ch'). The initial letter was dropped in the fourteenth century, so 'yichan' became 'ichan'. Incidentally, this has been proposed as the etymology of the viral disease chickenpox, which has nothing to do with chickens, or pox viruses (see page 242). Maybe it was originally 'ʒiccan pox'.

Numerous skin diseases can produce itching, from eczema to fungal infections, lice and insect bites. These have their own entries so I'll say no more about them here. Some serious illnesses such as liver, kidney and thyroid disease can also cause itching, and chronic itching can be a serious disease in its own right. Though formally defined as itching that lasts for six weeks or more, in reality it usually goes on for months or years and can lead to serious self-inflicted skin lesions from excessive scratching. The incessant itching and subsequent painful scratching can cause as much loss of quality of life as chronic pain, but unlike chronic pain there are no drugs available to alleviate it. Consequently, I'll confine myself to occasional, non-threatening itching without any underlying disease, technically called essential pruritus.

The most common reason for this is dry skin, which itself usually has an obvious cause: exposure to cold and dry weather, not drinking enough water, swimming in chlorinated pools and using harsh soaps and shampoos which strip moisturising oils from the skin. The simple answer is to stop doing these things and invest in some moisturiser.

But itches can arise without any obvious cause. To understand why, we need to go back in time again.

The medical definition of itch dates back to 1660, when the German doctor Samuel Hafenreffer described it as 'an unpleasant sensation that provokes the desire to scratch'.

For the next 337 years, biologists and medics itching to know more scratched away in vain. Itch sensations were known to travel up the same sensory neurons as pain, so itching was assumed to be a form of mild pain. But in 1997, biologists discovered a distinct type of itch sensor in the skin, which led to itching being reclassified as a distinct sensation, alongside four established ones: touch, temperature, body position and pain. This fifth sense was christened pruriception. Its function is to activate the scratch reflex, which dislodges parasites, biting and venomous insects, sticky or barbed plant material, irritants and dirt. This reflex is swift and powerful; next time you feel an itch, try to resist the temptation to scratch it.

Several types of pruriceptors are now known. Some are triggered by delicate touch, such as an insect landing on or creeping and crawling on the skin. But most are associated with immune cells such as mast cells, which secrete inflammatory compounds called histamines in response to contact with potential pathogens. As anyone who takes antihistamines to dampen down hayfever knows, histamines are very potent generators of itch, or prurigens. It seems likely – though not definite – that sudden itches with no apparent cause are a form of immune response to a potential invader.

This tight association between immunity and itching has seen the emergence of an interdisciplinary science called neuroimmune itch biology, which is dedicated to understanding the causes of itching and developing drugs to combat it. However, as a recent review of the state of the art admitted, 'there is much that remains unknown'.[16]

One of the unknowns is why itches move around. As we all know, an itch sometimes responds to being scratched by teleporting to a different place, often even itchier the second time around. This may be because the prurigen has been relocated by the act of scratching, or may have something to do with the social contagiousness of itching. People shown images or videos of other people scratching, or of itchy stimuli such as fleas and nettle rashes, respond by scratching themselves. In that respect itching is a bit like yawning, but in the case of itching there is at least a plausible explanation. Other people scratching is a warning that there are potential pathogens or irritants around and a bit of prophylactic scratching might be a good idea.

Even thinking about itchy things can cause an itch, which is maybe why itches proliferate and intensify. The initial itch-scratch reflex creates conscious awareness of itching, which leads to more itching in a vicious circle of itchy and scratchy.

One part of the body that is especially prone to itching, yet hard to scratch with dignity, is the anus. Anal itching is so common that it has its own name, pruritus ani. Like other forms of itch, it can be caused by an underlying skin condition or the use of harsh soaps. But one leading cause is poor anal hygiene, with traces of faeces and small wads of toilet paper irritating the sensitive skin around the anal opening. The solution is simple: don't be a dirty arsehole. There is a special circle of hell reserved for people like that.

Impetigo

Rather than drawing big red spots all over his face in a futile bid to get a day off school, maybe my son should have stuck some cornflakes to his chin instead. Then I might have been fooled into thinking he had impetigo, which is definitely a reason for a sick day.

Impetigo is a catch-all term for a bacterial attack on the skin (the word is derived from *impetre*, which is Latin for 'attack'). It usually announces itself with a rash of red sores or blisters which then burst, leaving yellow-brownish crusty scabs that look for all the world like cornflakes.

Impetigo usually gets a foothold on already-broken skin – a cut or insect bite, for example – but can then spread all over the body, and to other people. Picking at scabs is a major risk factor as mucky fingernails can introduce the causative bacteria – usually *Staphylococcus aureus* or *Streptococcus pyogenes* – directly into a wound. This is especially likely if the scab-picking is preceded by some nose-picking, as these bacteria often live harmlessly inside nostrils. This can make some people prone to repeated bouts of impetigo. Antibiotic nasal cream will root out the problem.

Antibiotic creams will also clear up impetigo, though non-antibiotic antiseptics are preferable for mild cases because of the risk of antibiotic overuse and resistance. Really bad outbreaks may need oral antibiotics. Doctors also advise keeping the lesions clean and dry and avoiding touching or scratching them. The scabs will eventually dry out and fall off. At which point children can go back to school, unless they know that trick with the cornflakes . . .

Rosacea

It is sometimes known as 'the curse of the Celts' because it appears to mostly afflict people with pale skin and has long been associated with getting sozzled. But rosacea is actually most common in women aged thirty to fifty, affects people of all ethnicities, and is just as likely to be caused by going running as by going to the pub.

The main symptom of rosacea – a pretty-sounding name for a rather unlovely condition – is ruddiness of the face, most often on the cheeks, forehead, chin and nose, and a stinging sensation when washing. At first the redness comes and goes, but over time becomes a permanent fixture. The red skin is often augmented by swelling, outbursts of pus-filled pimples, dilated capillaries across the cheeks and eventually, in some of the worst cases, bulbous enlargement of the nose. Even though women get it more frequently, men are more badly affected once it strikes.

The cause of rosacea is unknown, though there are many suggestions. One long-standing though unproven belief is that it is caused by drinking too much, too often. The association has some basis in fact: alcohol can make rosacea worse. But the causal link has not been established, at least for standard rosacea without the bulbous nose. According to the US National Rosacea Society, non-drinkers are just as likely to have the condition as drinkers.

The mythical association between rosacea and boozing goes back a long way. In his prologue to *The Canterbury Tales*, written around 1342 and appropriately set in a pub, Geoffrey Chaucer introduces us to the summoner, with his 'fyr-reed face', 'knobbes sittynge on his chekes' and love of 'drynken

strong wyn.' (If your Middle English is a bit rusty, this translates as 'red face, pimply cheeks and love of strong wine'. In
medieval England a summoner was a much-hated church
official who summoned people to appear before the eccle-
siastical courts for sins such as slander, usuary, tax-dodging
and witchcraft.) Shakespeare made the same mistake with
Bardolph, an associate of Falstaff who appears in four plays,
more than any other male Shakespearean character. He is a
habitual drunk with a bulbous red nose and ruddy cheeks. In
medieval France, rosacea was called *pustule de vin*, loosely
translated as 'wine zits'.

Another lurid but much more credible hypothesis points
the finger at tiny mites that live in our faces. These scaly,
eight-legged beasties are about a tenth of a millimetre long,
which mercifully makes them too small to be visible to the
naked eye. They feed on skin cells and sebum, an oily substance secreted by glands in the hair follicles. Humans – all
humans – are infested with them, mostly in facial areas but
also elsewhere on the body.

We host two species, *Demodex folliculorum* (which lives
in hair follicles) and *Demodex brevis* (which is slightly smaller
and lives inside the sebum glands). They spend their days
tucked away in their hidey-holes, but come out at night to
feed and have sex. On your face. But at least they don't poo
on you. Not until they die, at least. But we will come back
to that.

Also called follicle mites, *Demodex* are commonly called
eyelash mites, which tells you pretty much all you want to
know about their preferred habitat. Their formal name is
much more interesting, if a little mystifying. *Demodex* is a
mash-up of Ancient and Byzantine Greek words meaning
'lard-boring worm'. Lard refers to the fact that they eat
the waxy substance sebum, not a snarky comment about
their corpulence. They are not fat – if anything they are the
opposite, with an elongated body designed for squeezing into
narrow spaces. They are also not worms, and are definitely

not boring, in either sense of the word. The name, incidentally, was coined by the irascible anatomist Richard Owen, who for some reason is much better known for coming up with the word 'dinosaur' and founding the Natural History Museum in London.

Pluck out an eyelash or eyebrow hair and examine its root under a light microscope, and with luck you will meet your very own lardy boring worm.

Most people have about two mites per square centimetre of skin, but people with rosacea have been found to have up to twenty. This may be what causes the condition – the mites do not have an anus, so their faeces build up inside them and eventually kills them by bursting their abdomens (disgusting enough for you already?). The spilled faeces and exploded remains of its creator may trigger an inflammatory immune response.

Another possibility is that the mite infestation is caused by the rosacea, and not the other way round. The sebum of people who already have rosacea – which constitutes about 10 per cent of the population – may be especially nutritious and delicious, so the mites just scoff and breed like crazy. Intriguingly, however, the faeces of the mites contain a unique bacterium, *Bacillus oleronius*, which is wiped out by antibiotics that have also been shown to reduce the symptoms of rosacea. In other words, it probably isn't the mites living in our pores *per se* that are responsible. It is their crap.

Follicle lice infestations have also been linked to other skin problems, including the rosacea-like rash called demodicosis, the 'sandpaper skin' condition pityriasis folliculorum (see page 72 for more on flaky skin) and inflammation of the eyelids, a.k.a. blepharitis (see page 104).

Rosacea cannot be cured but is usually mild enough to be covered by cosmetics or soothed by skin creams. Bad cases can sometimes be brought under control by a course of antibiotics. Some people resort to a cosmetic procedure called

Intense Pulsed Light Therapy, which as its name suggests uses pulses of intense light to destroy damaged skin.

Even though the cause remains uncertain, there are some well-established factors that can trigger flare-ups in people who already have rosacea. These include sunburn (see page 309), heat, cold, hot drinks, caffeine, spicy food, cheese, stress, menopause and aerobic exercise such as running. And, of course, alcohol. Avoiding triggers can keep the symptoms in check.

The causal association between rosacea and alcohol may be spurious, but what of the bulbous red nose condition called rhinophyma, which often afflicts people with long-standing rosacea but is commonly seen as an indicator of over-fondness for the demon drink? Chaucer and Shakespeare clearly thought as much in the Middle Ages, but it wasn't until a bit later on – 2015, to be precise – that doctors finally got round to testing the idea scientifically. They interviewed fifty-two people with rhinophyma, and 150 without, about their drinking habits, and established that the condition is clearly associated with booze. The more people drank the more likely they were to have boozers' nose, and the boozier they were the bigger and ruddier their noses. You might say that the association was as plain as the noses on their faces.

The cause of rhinophyma – derived from the Greek for 'nose tumour', as in swelling rather than cancer – is a progressive and ultimately massive enlargement of the sebaceous glands on the nose, permanent dilation of blood vessels, and an immune response that causes the formation of granulomas, lumpy aggregates of white blood cells. The authors of the study point out that these changes are not often associated with rosacea. Untreated rosacea can lead to rhinophyma, but a more likely cause is getting your nose wet on a regular basis.

Chafing

In 2004, a pair of American dermatologists decided that it was time to get to the bottom of a painful condition that they kept on seeing in their clinics, especially among patients who were trying to get or stay fit by training for a marathon. They combed through records kept by medics at the Chicago marathon looking for case reports. From a total of 372 runners who presented at a first-aid station, they found that twenty of them were suffering from 'painful, erythematous and crusted erosions of the areola and nipples'.[17] In other words, jogger's nipple (erythematous is a technical way of saying 'red'). Some cases were so bad that the runners had bled through their shirts.

Jogger's nipple is a form of chafing, which is a painful but superficial skin injury caused by friction. Running for hours on end is a perfect recipe for it: repetitive motion, lots of sweat and fabric worn directly against the skin. This causes the upper layer of skin to separate slightly from the underlying tissue, leading to inflammation, soreness and, if the top layer is abraded away entirely, bleeding.

Nipples are especially vulnerable for obvious reasons, but other parts of the body can also chafe during a long run. The dermatologists looked into this too, and found that up to 16 per cent of marathon runners had a chafing injury after completing the race. Buttocks, bum cracks, thighs and groin areas were where most of the action was.

But you don't have to run 26.2 miles to get chafed. Anything that causes repetitive rubbing of the skin, especially in damp conditions, can do it. The bum crack is a hot spot as walking can cause skin-on-skin friction and the area is often quite sweaty – chafing is also known as 'sweat rash.' Being overweight or obese makes chafing more likely as there is more wobbly skin to rub against itself or clothing. A chafed bum crack can be severely debilitating.

The solution is to keep the area well ventilated, though with a certain nether region that is easier said than done. Where going naked is not possible, either keep the crack dry with talcum powder or antiperspirant, or lubricate it with Vaseline or something similarly slippery. There are products specially designed to prevent chafing of the arse crack. These anti-chafing gels dry quickly and leave what their manufacturers describe as a 'silky finish.' Smoooooth.

Chapped skin and lips

My mother-in-law has a theory about chapped lips: they did not exist before the invention of lip balm. Nobody had chapped lips when she was a child. But now everyone carries lip balm, and everybody has chapped lips. She hasn't quite gone as far as claiming that chapped lips were invented by Big Lipbalm to sell more product, but it is surely only a matter of time.

I suspect it is more a matter of selective memory. Lip balm was invented in the 1890s, which predates even my mother-in-law by some distance. A pharmacist called Charles Browne Fleet of Lynchburg, Virginia, set up a small business in his store selling patent medicines, balms and salves. One of his inventions was a stick of wax wrapped in foil to soothe chapped lips. He called it ChapStick. It flopped – his laxatives were much more in demand – and in 1912 he sold the recipe to a friend. Fleet was evidently a better inventor than salesman and, under new ownership and with a snazzy new logo, ChapStick flourished. It has been one of the biggest-selling lip balm brands in the US for more than 100 years and, like Hoovers, Post-it Notes, Sellotape and Bubble Wrap, so dominated the market that its trade name became generic.

Chapped lips are technically called cheilitis simplex, derived from the Greek for lip, *cheílos*, plus the fact that the cause is not complicated. It is what it looks like: excessive drying of the lips in hot and dry, or cold and dry, weather. Evaporation causes the skin of the lips – which is very thin and delicate to allow for their sensory and erotic functions – to dehydrate, flake and crack. Licking the lips – an almost impossible-to-resist temptation once chapping has started as it provides instant though temporary relief – just makes matters worse. The saliva evaporates, further drying the skin. Proteins in the saliva can also cause irritation of the fissures, leading to a vicious cycle of licking and cracking. Lip-licking can become a chronic habit. Really bad cases can progress to blistering and severe bleeding.

Other parts of the skin, notably hands and cheeks, can also dehydrate and chap, especially in the winter. The cause is the same – dehydration. Don't attempt to lick your cheeks. The word 'chap', incidentally, is of Middle English origin and means to split or burst.

Fortunately, the cure for chapping is simple: frequent application of a ChapStick (other lip balms are available) or hand cream. These contain barrier lubricants such as petroleum jelly, lanolin, palm wax or beeswax, which halt the evaporation of water from the lips, allowing rehydration and healing.

It doesn't make much difference which barrier lubricant the lip balm contains, though there is some evidence that lanolin – a wax extracted from sheep's wool – is better at promoting healing than petroleum jelly, though it often has a slightly ovine flavour. The NHS recommends petroleum jelly or beeswax. Some lip balms contain additives such as aroma and flavour compounds that may irritate the lips. They don't have any therapeutic value but just promote frequent application and hence sell more lip balms. But you're hardly going to break the bank buying lip balm. Find one you like and that works for you.

Nonetheless, lip balms are not without controversy. In 2015, the influential German consumer watchdog Stiftung Warentest – which roughly translates as 'Product Test Foundation' – advised people to avoid lip balms based on mineral oils such as petroleum jelly after it found they contain high levels of compounds classed as possibly carcinogenic. However, there is no scientific evidence of a link between lip balm and cancer.

Even less solid are rumours that lip balms contain substances designed to dry or abrade the lips – one brand supposedly contains finely ground glass – or even addictive drugs to get people hooked on balming. There is even an organisation called Lip Balm Anonymous which aims to help people break their addiction. These are conspiracy theories with no basis in fact. I have nonetheless alerted my mother-in-law.

Cuts and grazes

Some animals have amazing powers of regeneration. Lizards famously shed their tails to throw predators off their scent, and then grow a new one in a few weeks. Salamanders can regenerate entire limbs. Even some mammals can regenerate large body parts: red deer grow entirely new antlers every year.

We humans are not so lucky. We can regenerate a few millimetres of fingertip, and our livers also have miraculous powers of recuperation (phew!). But if we lose a limb, it has gone for good.

There is one area, however, where our bodies can do amazing repair work. Think of all those cut fingers, grazed elbows and barked shins. There may be a bit of scar tissue as a permanent reminder but on the whole you'd never know that you had once torn off skin, ripped open blood vessels, destroyed nerve endings, torn out hair follicles and gouged out connective tissues. This gory mess just cleans itself up and grows back.

Intuitively, wound healing might seem like a passive process. Skin is broken and bleeds, the blood clots to form a scab, and underneath it the normal processes of skin regeneration chug along as if nothing has happened, until the skin has regrown and the wound is healed.

But wound healing is actually a well-orchestrated sequence of events designed to rapidly plug the hole in the body's first line of defence and effect repairs.

The process is broken down into four stages: clotting, inflammation, proliferation and remodelling.

Blood clotting is a remarkable process that has arguably

saved more lives than any other function of the immune system. Unbroken skin is the body's first line of defence against pathogens and toxins, and as soon as it is breached, we are in peril.

If a wound is deep enough to bleed, even a tiny bit, then the damage has gone right through the epidermis – the dead outer layer of skin, which can take minor abrasions in its stride – and into the dermis, which is alive and contains nerves and blood capillaries. Any damaged blood vessels spill their contents into the wound, and the process of healing has already begun.

Step one is bleeding itself, technically called a haemorrhage, even if only a tiny amount of blood is spilt. This helps to flush debris and bacteria from the wound. That cleaning process can be helped by washing the wound in clean water and by sucking or licking the site of the wound, which is why these are instinctive responses to an injury.

But bleeding, sluicing, sucking and licking are not a long-term solution. So within seconds of the wound being inflicted, step two kicks in. First of all, the damaged blood vessels constrict to limit blood loss. And then the cavalry arrives.

Alongside red and white cells, human blood contains a third class of cell called platelets. These are small discs about a fifth the size of a red blood cell and a tenth as abundant. Their job is to be the 'sentinels of vascular integrity', as one research paper elegantly puts it.[18]

If a blood vessel is holed, passing platelets are attracted to the exposed dermis, migrate towards it and stick to it. They also become activated, sending out chemical calls for reinforcements. More platelets arrive and stick to the wound and to each other, and this process snowballs until the wound is plugged with platelets. Activated platelets also change shape, going from wrinkled spheres to something resembling a fried egg, in order to increase their surface area and plug the hole more efficiently.

Activated platelets also initiate a complex biochemical process called the coagulation cascade, which cements the nascent clot in place. They reverse the constriction of the patched-up blood vessel to allow circulating white blood cells and healing proteins to reach the injury. The most important of these proteins is fibrin. As its name suggests, it is fibrous and tough, and it forms a shell in and over the wound. Over the course of a few days, this dries, hardens and darkens into a tough dark-brown to black carapace that protects the wound from external threats and stops blood from leaking out. This is known as a scab. Think of it as a bit like a corrugated-iron shelter hastily thrown over a building with its roof blown off.

And like that roofless building, underneath the temporary covering, builders are beavering away. Their first job is to clear out any debris from the old roof. To that end the coagulation cascade also calls in white blood cells to clear out dead and damaged tissues and foreign bodies.

This marks stage two of the wound-healing process, inflammation. At this point the wound will be sore, inflamed and quite possibly oozing smelly pus through a fragile and still moist scab; the pus is the dead bodies of white blood cells that died on active duty. But after a couple of days the dirty work is done and healing can get underway in earnest.

During this stage we are often caught on the horns of a medical dilemma: to dress or not to dress (the wound, not ourselves)? Folk wisdom says to leave it undressed so 'it can breathe' and the 'air can get to it' and dry it out. As usual, folk wisdom is no match for medical science. Wounds heal better in a moist environment, shielded from contaminants. Nature's way of doing this is to form a scab. That takes time, but, in the meantime, nature can be mightily assisted by sticking a plaster on it.

However, think twice about applying antiseptics unless the wound is infected, as they can retard the healing process. Antiseptics are very effective at killing bacteria but many can also kill human cells called fibroblasts that are crucial members of the repair team. Over-the-counter antiseptics contain a wide variety of active ingredients, and the evidence for their effect on wound healing is patchy. Medical opinion is divided too.[19] But the NHS advises against using antiseptics on an uninfected wound as they generally do more harm than good. Clean water or saline solution are the best options to clean a recent wound and to keep it clean as it heals.

Stage three, proliferation, is when the repair team gets really busy. A new extracellular matrix is laid down, new blood vessels and nerves grow into it, and new skin cells migrate towards the base of the scab in a process called re-epithelialization. At the same time, specialist muscle cells called myofibroblasts pull the edges of the wound inwards to knit the new tissues together. All in all, it is a remarkable process of regeneration, though the tissue that grows back is often more fibrous and less flexible than the original. Full restoration comes later.

Once proliferation is complete – which takes at least a week and often more, depending on the depth and size of the wound – the scab is no longer needed and falls off. Unless its owner has already picked it off, which appears to be an almost irresistible temptation especially if the wound is itchy.

Itching is a good sign, caused by all that frenetic rebuilding stimulating itch receptors in and around the wounded skin. Thick and crusty old scabs can also cause itching directly.

Our instinct is to scratch and pick at the scab, but that is a bad idea. The repair process may not be complete, in which case you risk re-opening the wound and allowing bacteria to infect it. Scab-picking is a leading cause of the skin infection called impetigo (see page 78), characterised by painful yellow crusts that will make you want your scab back.

Once the wound has completely re-epithelialized, the final stage of wound healing, remodelling, kicks in. This is the long-term process of restoring the hastily reconstructed repair job to its former glory. It starts about three weeks after the injury and can go on for a year or more. The goal is to recreate the lost tissues in every last detail, from the positions of the blood vessels and nerves to the contours of the skin. But a full restoration is sometimes impossible and sections of the quick and dirty repair persist. These are known as scars. Wear them with pride, for they are mementoes of the human body's underappreciated powers of regeneration.

Sometimes, for reasons that are not clear, scar tissue can mount a hostile takeover of the surrounding skin. It is not unusual for scars to become thickened and raised over time, but these harmless hypertrophic scars occasionally just keep on going, overgrowing the site of the original injury. They sometimes originate from a very minor scar such as a healed acne spot, insect bite or ear piercing, or even erupt spontaneously on skin that has never been scarred at all.

These oversized scars are made of collagen and are called keloids; they are usually reddish-purple and are either firm and rubbery like a lump of old chewing gum, or shiny and fibrous like a lump of *very* old chewing gum. The word is derived from the Greek for 'hoof', *chílí*. They eventually stop growing and are not cancerous or infectious.

The cause of keloids is not known. They are more common in people with darker skin – there is no recorded case in anybody with albinism – and in people under thirty. They are mostly no bother though can become painful or itchy and are often unsightly. Surgical removal is an option.

Blisters

About thirty-five years ago, as a goth-curious teenager, I bought a pair of winklepickers in a shop in Gotham City, a.k.a. Leeds. I put them on straight away and walked around town all afternoon. By the time I went home I could barely walk. The shoes were narrow, stiff and ill-fitting and both of my heels were blistered to hell. But I resolutely soldiered on, determined to maintain my gothic cool. I had to wear my slippers to school the next day.

My blisters were technically called friction blisters. As the name suggests, these are caused by something hard and stiff, such as the back of a winklepicker, repeatedly rubbing against skin. This sets up a shear force between the dead outer layer of skin (epidermis) and the living inner layer (dermis). If the shear continues for long enough, the layers rip apart and fluid – usually the straw-coloured liquid called plasma, which is the watery component of blood – leaks into the space, causing the outer layer of skin to expand like a fluid-filled balloon.

Friction blisters can form on any part of the body but, for obvious reasons, are most common on the hands and feet. Especially the feet, as damp skin is more likely to shear and blister. Walkers, runners, gamers and soft-handed office workers who suddenly decide to pick up a shovel or sledge-hammer are especially at risk.

Friction blisters can form surprisingly quickly; just a few minutes of a repeated shear force is enough. It is a good idea to stop whatever is shearing the skin at this point, or the injury will progress from friction blister to burst blister. And if the first one hurts a lot, the second hurts a lotter.

As a bare minimum, apply a blister plaster, which is a dressing with a fluid-filled cavity almost exactly like a blister. This will take the brunt of the shear force and save your skin. Double-layered blister socks work the same way.

However painful a blister is, don't burst it. In fact, be grateful for the blister as the fluid protects the underlying skin from further damage and allows it to heal properly. The fluid and upper layer of stretched skin isn't the source of your pain; the underlying injury is. It will gradually wither and vanish as the skin heals.

If the damage also breaches a blood vessel, perhaps through a pinch injury such as trapping skin in a hinge, the result is a blood blister. These are distinct from bruises (see page 95) in that the spilled blood is contained within a blister rather diffused through the underlying tissue. As blood blisters heal, their contents congeal and dry up and end up rather like black pudding. Resist, if you can, the temptation to eat it.

Blisters can also be caused by burns and scalds which are bad enough to damage the dermis without breaching the epidermis. Ditto contact with corrosive chemicals and allergens such as the saliva of a mosquito (see page 263).

Some infectious diseases can also cause the skin to blister, the most common being chickenpox. In fact, the word 'blister' may be derived from the Old French *blostre*, which referred to skin nodules caused by leprosy. Talk about gothic horror.

Bruises and black eyes

As I write this, I am nursing a bruise on my hip, the result of tripping over while running and hitting the pavement about a week ago. It is quite a large bruise, and has progressed from a bluish colour to a mixture of sickly green and sickly yellow. If I squint at it, I can sort of make out a face. Actually, it is quite a thing of beauty.

Bruises are caused by blows – usually from a blunt instrument such as a pavement or fist – that are powerful enough to break blood vessels but not the skin. Blood leaks out of the ruptured capillaries and pools in the connective tissues under the surface, resulting in a reddish-purplish patch that can often be swollen and tender. The bruise, technically called a contusion, then ripens over days and weeks, progressing through a sequence of vivid colours then fading to nothing.

Bruises are classified according to size. Tiny ones less than 3 millimetres across are called petechiae; medium ones between 3 and 10 millimetres are purpurae; and anything over a centimetre is an ecchymosis. Eccky thump, you may be thinking, why so many names for something so simple? They may appear to have been invented to torment medical students, but they exist for a reason: the smaller bruises are sometimes associated with causes other than blunt trauma. Petechiae on the neck or face of a dead body, for example, are often taken as evidence of strangulation, while purpura can be a sign of bacterial meningitis. Neither are minor ailments, so enough said about both.

Bruises inflicted by a blow are almost always nothing to worry about; in certain circles they are a badge of honour. Players of the insanely violent sport roller derby frequently get massive bruises on their butts, which they take pictures of and post on Instagram with captions like 'Got a Really Beautiful Bruise on My Bum, Do You Want To See a Pic? It Has 12 Colours And Is the Size of My Head!'

Twelve colours is a bit of an exaggeration. There are actually four basic bruise colours. The first to appear is a bluish-purple, which is due to the oxygen-carrying pigment haemoglobin leaking out of red blood cells as they perish. The injured tissue is a low-oxygen environment so the haemoglobin is mostly in its deoxygenated state, which is bluish-purple and can appear black if the bruise is big enough. This is the classic 'black-and-blue' phase.

What happens next can be quite spectacular. The presence of inflammation and spilt blood causes white blood cells to rush to the site of the trauma to dispose of the bodies of their stricken red brethren. As well as gobbling up the remains, they also progressively break down haemoglobin into simpler and simpler molecules for recycling. The first degradation product is a pigment called biliverdin, which is bottle green. It is further degraded to the bright yellow bilirubin and finally the golden-brown hemosiderin, which is then cleared from the area by other white blood cells.

Different parts of the bruise can be at different stages of this sequence depending on how much blood there was to clear up in the first place, so a bruise can feature all of the colours (and mixtures thereof) at any one time. This constellation of coloured patches makes bruises fertile territory for pareidolia, the tendency to see meaningful patterns, especially faces, in inanimate objects. The face of Jesus is an especially common sight; He has been known to appear in the clouds, inside aubergines, on slices of burned toast or pancakes. One woman saw his face on a dumpling and sold it on eBay for $1,775. You may exclaim 'Jesus!' when you bang yourself, and lo! He sometimes appears. Bruises that look like Jesus are a common internet meme, though selling them on eBay is a challenge.

The entire process from black-and-blue to invisible can take three weeks or more to play out, and despite numerous folk remedies there is almost nothing you can do to speed it up. Sunlight can slightly accelerate the breakdown of bilirubin, but the bruise will essentially resolve at its own pace.

For some bruises that is a real bummer. The black eye is possibly the most noticeable form of bruising, closely followed by the love bite or hickey, caused by sucking skin hard enough to rupture the underlying capillaries. If your parents catch you with one of those, you really are cruising for a bruising.

Fat lips and head eggs

A blunt trauma can strike any part of the body, but when it hits the lips, the result really is swell. The lips are soft and stretchy and can balloon up alarmingly when a blow causes fluid to rush in. This swelling is called an angioedema but is commonly called 'fat lip'. Other squishy body parts such as the area around the eyes and the tongue can also double in size due to a blow. Allergic reactions can also cause dramatic swelling.

Another part of the body that is prone to dramatic swelling is the forehead. The skin covering the skull is very rich in blood vessels, which can leak a lot of fluid when damaged (and bleed profusely when the skin is broken). This fluid pools under the skin and forms an egg-shaped mass called, unsurprisingly, a head egg. The folk remedy for these is to smear them in butter. This is a waste of butter.

Both fat lips and head eggs look worse than they actually are, and should deflate of their own accord in a day or two. But blows to the head and allergic reactions can also be dangerous, so don't point and laugh too hard.

Calluses and corns

I once had a strangely heated argument with a girlfriend about the patches of hard skin on her feet. She was forever grinding them off with a pumice stone. I told her she should leave them alone because her feet were obviously growing thick skin to protect themselves from something. She laughed at me and said that she did not want ugly thick skin on her feet, but maybe I was into it? I got defensive; she made some withering remark about growing a thicker skin, and resumed her ruthless extirpation of her calluses. We split up soon afterwards.

Turns out I was right after all. I must call her to give her the good news! Calluses and their smaller relatives corns are natural protective responses to repeated skin friction. Calluses develop in response to external friction, such as using hand tools, wearing ill-fitting shoes, playing the guitar or writing with a pen. Corns are caused by internal friction when skin grinds in a circular pattern on underlying bones. They are largely harmless and actually quite helpful – calloused skin does not blister easily – but are ugly and can become infected and painful.

The word 'callus' comes from Latin for hard skin, which is also the source of the word 'callous'. I ought to have come back with a withering comment about my soon-to-be-ex's callous-ness, but I was too busy being an idiot.

Corns are so-called because they often resemble corn kernels in size, shape and colour. There is no clear dividing line between calluses and corns, but roughly speaking (geddit?) calluses are flat patches of hard skin and corns are raised lumps of hard skin. Or sometimes soft skin. Hard and soft corns are essentially the same thing but hard corns (also called 'durum', as in the hard wheat used to make pasta) arise on dry, flat skin and soft ones on moist, folded areas such as between the toes. Calluses can develop anywhere, but corns – also called clavi or helomata – tend to occur on the toes and fingers.

Both can be removed by abrasion, most efficiently after softening them with warm water. Corns can also be treated with corn plasters, which are circular pieces of sticky, absorbent felt infused with salicylic acid, which cushion the corn and gradually erode it. But unless the root cause of the corn is not addressed, they just come back. Unlike me in that pathetic argument. I'm so over it!

A few other conditions cause annoying but largely harmless lumps to appear on the skin. One very common one is keratosis pilaris (KP), which affects up to 70 per cent of adolescents and 40 per cent of adults. The name means 'keratinised hair follicles', which is exactly what it is. Hair follicles on the upper arms and thighs become plugged with the structural protein keratin, which is the principal component of hair and nails (and rhino horn) and also toughens up the outer layer of skin. The result is small, pale, horny bumps that look a bit like small goose pimples – it is sometimes called 'chicken skin' – but feel rough to the touch and don't go down. They occasionally itch.

KP comes and goes – some people find it improves in warmer weather, which may have something to do with exposing the skin to sunshine. Or maybe not; the cause is unknown. My younger son has it on his upper arms; he says it gets worse when he eats bread so my older son dubbed it 'bread arm' to annoy him, which worked a treat. However, there is no established link to eating bread. In fact, it is so common and harmless that calling it a skin condition at all is questionable.

KP is also called 'lichen pilaris'. In this context lichen does not refer to the slow-growing fungus-like organisms that grow on the surface of rocks and trees, but to a skin condition characterised by small, hard, circular patches that look a bit like, er, lichens.

There is also lichen planus, which means 'flat lichen'. It produces a rash of shiny, raised, reddish-purple blotches on the skin, and sometimes inside the mouth. The lesions may be criss-crossed with fine white lines; they sometimes itch but are otherwise harmless. The cause of them is not known, but it seems to be an immune response to something or other. Up to 1 per cent of people have it at any one time. It usually clears up on its own in a few months.

Styes, chalazia, blepharitis and conjunctivitis

If pustules on the rim of the nose are inordinately painful, the ones we get on the edges of our eyelids are absolute agony. Technically called a hordeolum but commonly known as a stye, they can arise very suddenly and promise a week or two of ugliness, swelling and pain. They often look a bit like zits, with a pus-filled head surrounded by red and swollen skin. That is because, to all intents and purposes, they are zits (see page 60). Both are caused by an infected oil-producing gland, often inside a hair follicle. In the case of styes, this follicle contains an eyelash. And also a sebum-secreting gland called the gland of Zeis, named after the German ophthalmologist and surgeon Eduard Zeis, who also coined the term 'plastic surgery'.

These glands can become blocked by dirt or dead skin, which creates a nice buffet for bacteria. If the bacteria – almost invariably the pesky *Staphylococcus aureus*, which also causes impetigo – gain the upper hand, the whole follicle can become the site of a pitched battle between them and our immune system. The result: an inflamed and pus-filled pit of hell.

As well as these external (or Zeisian) styes, there are also internal ones that arise from the infection of a different type of gland on the inside of the eyelid. These meibomian glands – also named after a German doctor, Johann Heinrich Meibom – produce an oily and comically-named substance called meibum which helps to prevent the surface of the eye from drying out. They, too, can become blocked and infected.

There are twice as many glands in the upper eyelid than in the lower, so internal styes are more common upstairs than downstairs.

The best way to avoid styes is eyelid hygiene. Gently clean the edges of eyes each morning using a warm, moist flannel or cotton bud dipped in warm water (no soap!). This will clear away any dangerous gubbins and the warmth will help to keep the sebum inside the eyelash follicle liquid and hence mitigate against blockages. Avoid touching the eyes with unwashed fingers (like, who does that anyway these days?!). But no amount of cleanliness can totally prevent styes, so don't beat yourself up when you get one.

And don't beat the stye up either. As with a zit, relief can be found by bursting the pustule. But doctors strongly advise against this, as infectious pus can leak into other eyelash follicles or meibomian glands and set off a chain reaction. One stye is misfortune enough; two or three at once starts to look like carelessness. There is also the risk of lancing the eyeball rather than the stye. Medical advice is to lump it. Warm compresses and non-steroidal anti-inflammatory painkillers (i.e. not aspirin) can ease the swelling and pain. Avoid eye makeup even if you really need it in the circumstances and don't wear contact lenses. Styes usually clear up by themselves in a week or two.

The word, incidentally, has no connection to the mucky little houses that pigs live in, but comes from the Old English word for 'rise'. Hordeolum is from the Latin for 'barley', presumably because the size and shape resemble a barleycorn.

Sometimes an internal stye can progress to a chalazion, which is a large and hard, though often painless, lump under the eyelid. It is basically a super-stye caused by a chronically blocked meibomian gland; they are also known as meibomian cysts. The lump is congealed meibum trapped inside the blocked gland. The word is derived from the Ancient Greek for 'hailstone', which neatly describes their size (variable) and hardness (very).

The gland does not always become infected, so chalazia can sometimes form without passing through the internal stye phase first. They can become so big that they press on the eyeball and distort vision. They usually clear up by themselves but occasionally need to be professionally lanced and drained.

Chalazia are often a complication of blepharitis, or chronic inflammation of the eyelids, which can lead to redness, itchiness, soreness, scaliness and crustiness. Blepharitis can be caused by bacterial infections, eczema (see page 68), infestations of tiny, horrible mites that live in eyelash follicles (see page 80), or allergies, but also by partially blocked meibomian glands. Around half of people seen by opticians have it. The answer, again, is good eyelid hygiene.

Another risk of mucky eyes is conjunctivitis, which is a kind of all-purpose inflammation of the eyes. It is often called red eye or pink eye because of what it does to the white parts of the eyeball (sclera). Technically, it is an inflammation of the conjunctiva, the tissue that covers the sclera and lines the eyelids. As well as turning the eyes pink or red it can make them itchy, gritty, watery and sticky. It is often a sign of infection but can be caused by allergies.

Infectious conjunctivitis is most often viral, so antibiotic eye drops won't help to clear it up though may soothe the grittiness. Cool compresses can also help.

But prevention is always better than cure. So if you don't want styes, chalazia, blepharitis or red eyes, the answer is to keep your eyes clean. Or, as a wag might say, don't let your eyelids turn into a pigsty.*

---

* The words have totally different origins, but a pun is a pun.

Twitchy eyelids

ural and drive you to distraction and so on, all of which makes things that bit worse. The twitching keeps going even during sleep but being the twitching keeps stops — usually within a week — you're down twitching all by itself.

In popular culture, twitchy eyelids are often a signifier of madness. Think of Chief Inspector Dreyfus in the *Pink Panther* movies, his eyelid spasming furiously as he is driven up the wall by the nincompoop Inspector Clouseau. In real life, twitchy eyelids are a signifier of nothing much at all. Most people get one from time to time, suddenly and for no apparent reason, which stops all by itself just as suddenly and mysteriously after a day or two.

Most cases of twitchy eyelid are a disorder called myo-kymia (Greek for 'muscle wave'), which for unknown reasons triggers a muscle or group of muscles to quiver involuntarily. This usually manifests as a wave-like rippling on the surface of the skin, but in eyelids it merely causes twitching, usually of the lower lid but sometimes the upper. To the twitcher it feels like a spasm of Dreyfus-like proportions, but it is rarely visible to other people.

Doctors are generally unconcerned by twitchy eyelids as they usually clear up by themselves and can't be treated anyway. There is a more serious condition called blepharo-spasm which also comes and goes for no apparent reason but gets progressively worse, so if you are bothered by frequent and escalating eyelid twitching, or have had twitching for more than two weeks, it is wise to get it checked out.

Many causes have been suggested for myokymia, includ-ing stress, anxiety, too much caffeine, too much alcohol, dehydration and tiredness. In other words, life. Doctors might recommend rest and a warm compress to the eye, and advise you to avoid those triggers. Above all, don't worry about your twitchy eyelid, as this will stress you, make you tired and drive you to caffeine and/or alcohol. Like most minor ailments, it will go away all by itself. But while the twitching goes on – and it can go on and on, sometimes lasting two weeks – it will drive you as mad as Dreyfus.

Hard as nails

Your eyes may be windows on the soul. But if you want a window on something more down to earth, try the big and horny slabs of keratin on the ends of your toes and fingers. Many diseases, both harmless and harmful, can produce tell-tale changes to your nails. They can change shape, change colour, grow in the wrong direction and sometimes fall off.

Just like the rest of the body, nails are vulnerable to injuries and infections. The anatomy of a nail is quite complex and creates numerous opportunities for damage to occur, and/or pathogens to get in. One especially delicate area is the nail fold, which is the skin around the edge of the nail itself. It can be damaged or torn quite easily, leading to a hangnail – actually a hanging piece of skin, not nail. They are painful and can become infected with bacteria, leading to a painful condition called paronychia. Nail-biters are especially prone to it.

Nails can also become infected with fungi (see page 253) and are sometimes their own worst enemy, growing in the wrong direction and burrowing painfully down into the nail folds. Ingrowing nails (see page 29) are much more common on toes than fingers, which has led to the finger (or toe) being pointed at ill-fitting shoes.

Nails also turn black from time to time, usually as the result of a hard blow, say being hit with a hammer or having something heavy dropped on them. This can burst blood vessels under the nail and lead to a subungual hematoma – essentially a bruise. (Subungual means 'under the nail'; ungual is a zoological word meaning 'hoof', 'claw' or 'nail', as in ungulate.) The blood can create painful pressure that needs to be relieved by drilling into the nail. Minor blows can cause much smaller, long and thin bruises called splinter haemorrhages.

The hematoma starts off deep red then darkens to black. It can also cycle through the green-to-yellow-to-amber colour changes seen in normal bruising under the skin (see page 96). If the injury is severe enough, the whole nail eventually dies and falls off and a replacement grows up from the nail bed. Nails grow very slowly – about a tenth of a millimetre a day for fingernails and half that for toenails – so it can take six months to completely regrow a fingernail and up to eighteen months for a big toenail.

Fingernails serve to both protect the delicate finger ends and help with fine motor control by giving the fingertip something hard to push against when it touches something. So being without a fingernail for a few months is not ideal. Concentrate when hammering nails into walls.

Nails can also be darkened by a totally harmless condition called melanonychia, which is when one or more streaks of the dark brown pigment melanin grow up from the nail bed. This is more common in dark-skinned people but can happen to almost anyone. It is totally normal but if it persists for months without growing out it is worth getting it checked as it looks very similar to a rare form of cancer called subungual melanoma.

Nails also often feature small white spots called leukonychia. Again, these are almost always harmless, caused by minor injuries to the nail root – the part of the nail under the skin where new nail grows from. Ridges are also common and generally harmless. Horizontal ones – called Beau's lines after a French doctor called Dr Beau who described them in 1846 and hence earned himself a rather minor form of medical immortality – are the legacy of a period of reduced nail growth due to illness, injury or malnutrition. By the time they creep out from under the cuticle, whatever it was that caused them has probably passed. Vertical lines and ridges are also common. They are almost always a harmless consequence of getting older: your nails can get wrinkly too. If they bother you, an emery board will see them off.

But some changes to the nails can indicate an underlying medical condition that requires attention. Muehrcke's lines – named after an American doctor, Dr Muehrcke – are bands of pale colouration running horizontally across the fingernails reminiscent of the hooped cherry-and-white shirts worn by Wigan Warriors Rugby League Club. They can be a symptom of hypoalbuminemia, a protein deficiency caused by liver, kidney or gastrointestinal disease. Mees' lines – named after a Dutch doctor called, you guessed it, Dr Mees – are very similar and can indicate heavy metal poisoning or kidney disease. If you ever need to distinguish a Muehrcke's line from a Mees' line, there is a rule of thumb. Literally. Muehrcke's lines only appear on fingernails. Mees' lines also appear on the thumbnails (and toenails).

There are various other nail discolorations and deformations that can be a warning sign of all manner of conditions. Brittle or fraying nails may be caused by vitamin or mineral deficiencies, thyroid problems or kidney disease. Very thick or very red nails can indicate heart problems. Yellow nail beds can be a sign of diabetes or liver disease. Lifted nails, where the nail detaches from the nail bed, can result from infections or over-zealous manicures; the detached nail turns pale and occasionally green if it becomes infected. Nails that grow down over the fingertips (clubbing) or up (spooning) are indicative of malnutrition, kidney, liver or cardiovascular disease.

I bet you are looking at your nails right now.

Chilblains

My dear, departed grandma was a fan of the 'improving walk', which usually meant dragging me and my big sister across some godforsaken and frigid Lancashire wasteland. When we got home, she would scold us for holding our frozen hands and feet too close to the fire. 'You'll get chilblains,' she would say.

'What are chilblains?' we'd ask.

'They're what you get if you hold your cold hands and feet too close to the fire.'

I never found out what chilblains are, and I don't think my grandmother actually knew. I dismissed them as some forgotten malady of the Victorian slums; even their name (a contraction of 'chill' and 'blain', an archaic word for a sore) screamed 'anachronism'. This suspicion was confirmed when I read *Jane Eyre*, who suffered from them during winter at her horrible school for orphaned girls. 'Our clothing was insufficient to protect us from the severe cold: we had no boots, the snow got into our shoes and melted there: our ungloved hands became numbed and covered with chilblains, as were our feet.'

I ignored my grandmother's warnings and defiantly held my hands near to the fire. Whatever chilblains were, I wasn't going to get one.

My grandma died years ago, as did the memory of her warnings. And then I read about one of the rarer symptoms of Covid-19. Doctors reported being inundated with patients complaining of painful swellings on their toes, ankles and feet. When dermatologists examined them, they made a surprising diagnosis: chilblains.

I now accept that chilblains exist. I also know why, despite my reckless toasting, I didn't succumb. Some people are prone to chilblains, others aren't. I guess I'm just one of the lucky ones.

My grandma also turned out to be right about holding your hands too close to the fire. Chilblains are caused by rapid warming of cold extremities – fingers, toes, earlobes and noses. When we get cold, blood is withdrawn from these peripheral areas to prevent chilled blood from flowing back to vital internal organs; extremities are considered worth sacrificing for the greater good.

Blood is shut out by closure of the tiny blood vessels called capillaries. This temporary bloodlessness is why fingers and toes can go very pale or even blue when you get really cold. They also go numb, which is caused by sensory nerves shutting down due to lack of oxygen.

Some people are extremely prone to 'dead finger', with entire fingers or hands turning ghostly and waxy white after the briefest contact with cold. Even taking something out of the freezer can trigger it. This is called Raynaud's syndrome and it affects about one in twenty people. It is almost always harmless but can also be a symptom of a serious underlying condition, including atherosclerosis and rheumatoid arthritis. As always, if it is very bad or getting worse, see a doctor. Prolonged and severe attacks can cause the tissues to die and gangrene to set in.

The syndrome is named after a 28-year-old French medical student called Maurice Raynaud, who described it in his 1862 doctoral thesis. Raynaud observed that the process was characterised by a sequence of colour changes: pink to white (bear in mind that all of his patients were white-skinned), white to blue, and blue to red. The first is caused by the withdrawal of blood; the second by blood trickling back in but being greedily de-oxygenated by oxygen-starved cells, turning red haemoglobin into blue deoxyhaemoglobin; the third by a transient increase in blood flow to compensate for a period without it, called a reactive hyperaemia. This is often accompanied by tingling, pins and needles or pain, which is a symptom of the capillaries rapidly reopening and sensory nerves coming back online.

This is also what causes chilblains. If the capillaries reopen too quickly – say, because you are warming your frozen fingers on the fire – the inrushing blood can damage the vessels, causing temporary swelling, redness, pain, itching and burning. Chilblains clear up by themselves and are easily avoided by staying warm, or at least not warming up your frozen extremities too quickly. Exactly why SARS-CoV-2 does the same remains an unsolved mystery.

Unsurprisingly, people with Raynaud's syndrome are also prone to chilblains.

Raynaud's thesis describing a new disease won him his doctorate and must have felt like the start of a brilliant career, but it was actually a high point. He worked in various hospitals in Paris but never managed a senior appointment, and dropped dead suddenly aged forty-six. He did not even live to see his name in lights: the term Raynaud's syndrome did not enter the medical literature until the 1890s.

Burns and scalds

Every now and then my wife can be seen at the kitchen sink wrapping cling film around a finger while running it under the cold tap. This is a sure-fire sign that she has burned or scalded herself while cooking or making a cup of tea. Her finger ends up looking like a cling film-wrapped mummy, often for days afterwards. She says it helps the wound to heal. She is, at best, half right.

Burns and scalds – collectively called thermal injuries – are among the most painful but least interesting ways we can injure our skin. The heat simply cooks the tissue, which then slowly repairs itself in the same way as after cuts and grazes (see page 88).

The manner of cooking varies according to the heat source. Flesh can be flame-grilled, toasted, broiled, boiled, steamed or even fried. I once carelessly splashed hot cooking oil onto the knuckle of my index finger, and I can tell you that a shallow-fried finger hurts a lot. And also smells like frying bacon. I did not suck my finger as I am vegetarian, and definitely not a cannibal.

The degree of burning depends on the depth of damage to the skin, which is determined by how hot the heat source was and how long it was in contact. First-degree burns/scalds are confined to the already-dead outer layer of skin, or epidermis. They are sore but do not blister, remain dry, and heal in as little as five days. They generally don't need medical attention unless they become infected.

Burns or scalds that penetrate into the dermis, the living layer of skin under the epidermis, are classed as second-degree. These are further divided into superficial and deep;

superficial burns are red, blistered, moist and very painful and take two to three weeks to heal, but can often be dealt with at home using first aid. Deep burns are yellow or white, dry and often blister-free, and paradoxically less painful as sensory nerves are destroyed. They need specialist medical attention and sometimes do not heal without skin grafts.

Third- and fourth-degree burns are . . . well, you really don't want to know.

The briefest encounter with a flame, hot pan, hot oil, steam or boiling water will damage skin, but even relatively cool temperatures can still do some harm. Water at 60°C – the upper allowable limit of domestic hot water heaters, as set out in the International Plumbing Code (section 501.6, if you want to check) – is scalding if the contact exceeds three seconds, and water at 50°C will scald after a minute or two. For comparison, a hot bath is about 40°C and candle wax melts at about 50°C.

Burns can also be inflicted by contact with very cold things, such as ice cubes or metal. These can freeze the water inside skin cells, forming ice crystals that kill and damage the tissues. An ice burn usually turns white and fails to tingle as it warms up; bad ones can freeze through the epidermis and blister like a thermal burn. Mouths and tongues are especially susceptible as they often come into contact with ice in the form of cubes and lollies. The lolly-stuck-to-the-tongue thing is not an urban myth – a very cold lolly can freeze a layer of saliva between itself and the tongue. If this happens, it is best to let the warmth of the tongue gently melt the lolly away rather than yanking it off, which can add insult to injury by tearing off skin. Avoid the temptation to lick metal poles in winter.

Scalding with steam is often worse than with boiling water for reasons you probably learned in chemistry class. Both are roughly at 100°C (depending on the altitude and how pure the water is) but steam also packs the extra punch of what physical chemists call the latent heat of condensation. This is an extra injection of energy that water molecules at boiling point need to get over the line and actually evaporate from the liquid phase into the gas phase. Water molecules in the gas phase – collectively called steam – carry this extra energy around as they whizz through the air. When steam condenses back to water, perhaps by coming into contact with a surface cooler than itself, such as human skin, it dumps the latent heat onto the surface. In the case of water, the latent heat of condensation is about 2,250 kilojoules per kilogram. That is actually more than the thermal energy contained in a kilogram of liquid water at 100°C, which is about 420 kilojoules. So steam is much more scaldy than hot water.

The words 'scald' and 'scold', incidentally, mean similar things but have totally different origins. Scald comes from *ex calidus*, Latin for 'from hot'. Scold is derived from the Old Norse *skáld*, meaning, weirdly, 'poet'.

Recommended first-aid for burns and scalds is to run the affected area under cool or lukewarm water for twenty minutes – avoid very cold or iced water, or bags of frozen peas, as they can damage the skin further. The cool water carries residual heat away from the burn and soothes and cleans the wound. After that, wrap the injury loosely in a single layer of cling film. Really. The film is sterile and so protects the wound from getting infected, and is also see-through so you or a doctor can see the damage without removing the film. But don't wrap it tightly as the burned area may swell or blister.

Cling film is a stopgap and should be removed once the wound has been medically assessed, or you decide that it is not bad enough to seek help. After that it is a waiting game. The wound should be dressed with a light gauze or plaster because, contrary to folk wisdom, wounds do not heal better or faster if exposed to air. Moist environments with some protection from contaminants are ideal for burn healing. This is why those painful burns sustained to the roof of the mouth from hot food or drink heal so rapidly.

Doctors advise against applying antiseptic and other creams unless the wound shows signs of becoming infected, as they can retard the natural healing process and inflict further damage. They also strongly advise against another folk remedy, butter, as there is no evidence that it soothes the wound or helps it heal. Cover the burn, take a painkiller, and let nature do its work.

Splinters

When I was nine years old, my dad went to Ghana to do some fieldwork – he was a biologist who had chosen a type of fern called bracken as his specialist subject, mainly because it grows all over the world and he likes to travel to exotic locations. While he was there, the military staged a coup d'état, he was arrested at gunpoint for birdwatching near an army base and he almost cut off his own finger after mistakenly believing he had been bitten by a deadly Gaboon viper. But the thing that left the most lasting impression on him was getting a really nasty splinter.

One day, while working in the forest, he jabbed his hand into some undergrowth (always a good idea in the tropics) and speared the fleshy flap between his thumb and forefinger on a pointy rattan cane. The tip snapped off and left a big, barbed sliver of wood in the flesh. He couldn't get it out so just put a plaster on it and carried on. He brought it home and it stayed in his hand for years; he used to let me and my sister feel it. Eventually, he had it surgically removed.

As splinters go, that was a whopper. They are usually no more than tiny slivers of wood, glass or some other material that penetrate the outer layer of skin and settle in the layers beneath. But they punch well above their weight in terms of pain.

Dermatologists classify splinters into two types: biological and non-biological. The classic wooden splinter, which is usually caused by walking barefoot or rubbing a hand over, erm, some splintered wood – is a biological one, as are cactus barbs, sea urchin spines (another thing my dad has personal experience of, see page 279) and bone splinters.

Non-biological ones include shards of glass, plastic, fibre-glass, metal and pencil graphite. Whichever visionary came up with that classification probably deserves the Nobel Prize in Stating the Bleeding Obvious.

Dermatologists also recommend removing splinters as soon as possible, using sterilised needles and tweezers. Again, visionary stuff. Splinters are not usually dangerous – there are a few case studies of large splinters penetrating vital organs, which begs the question of the upper size limit of a splinter – but can introduce bacteria and other gubbins into the wound, often raising a painful inflammatory response. An unremoved splinter can become surrounded by sore, inflamed and pus-filled tissue as the immune system battles gamely to defeat what to it is a vast chunk of foreign matter. Unreachable splinters eventually work themselves out through the natural cycle of skin shedding and renewal.

For obvious reasons, splinters are most common on the hands and feet. But nowhere is safe. Just ask my younger son, who once shinned up a metal pole in the school playground and slid back down, only to receive a metal splinter in a delicate part of his anatomy that I will spare you the details of, except to say that the offending pole became known as the 'scrotum pole'. I think my family deserves some sort of prize as World Splinter Champions.

Varicose veins

My mum always blames me for the varicose veins on her leg, which is a bit unfair. She bases this on the fact that they first appeared when she was pregnant with me, which was (a) ages ago, and (b) hardly my fault. But pregnancy is a recognised cause of varicose veins, so I will reluctantly accept responsibility. Sorry about your horrible veins, Mum.

Varicose veins are swollen and often bulgy blood vessels, often dark blue or purple in colour. They usually appear on the legs and ankles but can be found pretty much anywhere (full disclosure: I have a small patch on my left buttock which I thought was a bruise until it didn't go away. God knows what caused it; I blame my mother). They are unsightly but usually harmless, though sometimes cause discomfort and need to be treated.

Varicose veins also occur inside the anus, though thankfully not mine. In this location they are called haemorrhoids (see page 214).

Technically there are three types: the classic 'trunk' varicose veins which are thick, long, lumpen and bulbous; reticular varicose veins, which are thinner and flatter and form a wiggly network like the veins in a red Windsor cheese; and telangiectasia varicose veins, which are very small clusters of red, thread-like veins that often crop up on the face. Telangiectasia is a mash-up of the Ancient Greek words for 'end', 'vessel' and 'stretched'. They are also known as spider veins because of their web-like appearance.

The cause of all three types is dodgy valves. Veins – which are the vessels carrying de-oxygenated blood back to the heart – are lined with valves to keep the blood flowing in the right direction. Blood pressure in the veins is much lower than in the arteries, so the blood tends to pool or even backtrack. The valves stop this from getting out of control.

To see a venous valve in action, locate a vein on your forearm. Press down on it with the index and middle finger and then, keeping the middle finger in place, slide the index finger towards the elbow to squeeze to evacuate a section about 5 centimetres long. If you keep your middle finger pressed down the vessel will not refill with blood, because the valve prevents backflow. Release the finger and the vein quickly fills up with blood flowing towards the heart.

The value of these valves can be appreciated by looking at a varicose vein. When the valves fail, the blood pools and backs up, causing the vessels to dilate or partially rupture. Exactly what causes the valves to weaken or malfunction is not known but there are some well-established risk factors. People who are old, fat, pregnant or spend a lot of time standing up are especially prone. They run in families, which is why I blame my mother for the patch of reticular varicose veins on my buttock.

'Varicose veins' is one of those terms, like PIN number or Lake Windermere, which contains a superfluous word. Varicose means 'with dilated veins' in Latin, so when we say 'varicose veins' we are actually saying 'with dilated veins veins'. But that is another argument I will never win.

Treatment is rarely necessary, though some people find that the varicose veins in their legs and ankles ache, throb, swell up or itch. This can often be treated with compression socks or by resting up with the affected leg elevated. But occasionally the offending veins have to be destroyed. This is usually done by injecting a type of expanding foam into the vein which causes it to swell up even more and rupture. The body naturally re-routes the venous blood and the now-abandoned vein eventually withers and degrades. If that does not work, the treatment of last resort is called ligation and stripping, which requires surgery. The vein is tied off either side of the varicose section (ligation) and then yanked out with forceps (stripping).

Some people choose to have their varicose veins done for cosmetic reasons. Mum, if this book is a success, I will pay for you to have it.

Stretch marks and cellulite

Another skin condition associated with pregnancy is stretch marks. Technically called striae distensae ('extended streaks' in Latin) they are indeed stretch marks: scars left from damage to the skin caused by it being rapidly stretched. Pregnancy is the most common cause but adolescents who shoot up (as in, grow fast, not as in inject drugs) and body-builders can also get them. They are harmless and usually fade with time.

Women also account for the vast majority of cases of cellulite, a mysterious condition characterised by dimpling of the skin around the buttocks, thighs and abdomen. It is also called orange-peel skin. The cause is unknown, but skin with a lot of subcutaneous fat beneath it is more likely to dimple. There is no proven treatment. It is harmless but considered unsightly, though is so common that it should probably be considered entirely normal.

Dark circles

Back in the day, when sleeping was for wimps and bloodshot, dark-circled and puffy eyes were an occupational hazard of being young rather than being old, my wife used to keep a regular supply of a product that claimed to make tired eyes look as fresh as a daisy. For reasons lost in the mists of time, it became known in our family as 'boogly eye gel'. Her mother decided that she was in need of some, went to the cosmetics shop that stocked it . . . and asked for a tube of boogly eye gel. We like to remind her of this.

I'm not sure if it even worked, but we could all use some of that ol' boogly magic from time to time. Who hasn't looked in the mirror after a heavy or sleepless night – boogly nights, if you will – and shuddered at the sight of the eyes staring back?

These tell-tale signs of debauchery are actually there all the time, but are usually invisible. Bloodshot eyes are caused by dilation of the blood vessels in the cornea, often because not getting enough shut-eye – literally having your eyes open for too long – can induce mild inflammation. The blood vessels are always there but usually go unnoticed.

Ditto the dark circles. The skin around the eyes is thin and delicate and anything that makes it pallid, such as being tired or hungover, renders it slightly more translucent than usual. The darkness is actually just the blood vessels and underlying tissues showing through. An early, sober night should sort it out; failing that, wear some makeup. Cucumbers and tea bags are not totally useless, as we shall see.

Bags under the eyes are not only a consequence of tiredness and high living, but also of laziness. They are a sign of the build-up of fluid in the tissues around the eyes, technically known as periorbital edema. The simplest cause is merely a redistribution of bodily fluids from lying horizontal, which is why eyes are often puffy after waking up, and can be especially so after a really long kip.

Lack of sleep can do the same, but for different reasons. Sleep deprivation disrupts the delicate system of fluid balance controlled by the kidneys and leads to fluid retention. Some of that fluid ends up under the eyes and swells the tissue. Too much salt is another cause of fluid retention. Alcohol, by contrast, causes dehydration, but still makes eyes puffy because it disrupts sleep. Puffy eyes can make dark circles appear even darker by casting shadows under the eyes.

Again, eye puffiness will usually go away by itself after a decent night's sleep, but if you need a quick remedy a cold compress made from ice cubes wrapped in a flannel will also help. Putting slices of cool cucumber or used tea bags (cold) onto the eye sockets does the same; boogly eye gel is also cooling, though there is no decent scientific evidence that it does anything. The oft-repeated claim that cucumbers contain vitamins and nutrients that infuse into the skin around the eyes and rejuvenate it is total vegetables.

Dark, puffy eyes can be caused by underlying conditions such as anaemia and allergies, but are usually nothing to worry about. Ageing also makes them worse as the skin loses its elasticity and becomes prone to sagging.

Humans are finely attuned to facial appearance – we have a brain region called the fusiform face area whose sole function is to recognise and interpret faces – and research shows that we quickly and effortlessly spot the signs of sleep deprivation, mainly from the eyes. This may have consequences, for example in the workplace where bosses could discriminate against tired-looking employees. People who appear tired are also rated as less attractive than when they don't, and one of the main goals of cosmetic surgery is to reduce the appearance of tiredness. That is a bit drastic; pass the boogly eye gel.

Pallor and waxy complexion

'Thou cream-faced loon! Where got'st thou that goose look?' Macbeth, the usurper king of Scotland, is already in a bit of a funk about his increasingly desperate situation when a servant, pale and goose-pimpled with fear, comes in to tell him that an army of 10,000 soldiers is preparing to attack. Macbeth gives him both barrels: 'Go prick thy face, and over-red thy fear, thou lily-liver'd boy. What soldiers, patch? Death of thy soul! Those linen cheeks of thine are counsellors to fear. What soldiers, whey-face?'

Shakespeare knew that pallid skin conveys extreme fear. But it is also a symptom of numerous other unpleasant states, both small and large – emotional trauma, infections, sleep deprivation, nausea, nutrient deficiencies, anaemia and low blood sugar.

The underlying problem is always the same: a reduction of oxygenated blood flowing to the skin, either because there is less of it or it is needed more urgently elsewhere.

Macbeth's unfortunate servant was in fear, both for his life and of his tyrannical master, and so his body had initiated its 'fight-or-flight' response. One element of that is to withdraw blood from the periphery to the muscles where it might be needed for fighting or running away. Hence his cream/linen/whey-coloured face.

Under extreme duress that creamy complexion can shade to a sickly green. This happens when oxygenation declines further and the dominant colour of blood in capillaries under the skin is the blue of deoxygenated haemoglobin. Under pale yellowish skin this can meld to green. Extreme nausea, for example, both initiates the fight-or-flight response and causes breathing to shallow as the body dedicates its resources to preparing for a hurl (see page 192).

Low blood sugar makes us pale because the body withdraws blood from the periphery, which it calculates can be sacrificed for the greater good, to the internal organs, which are too important to fail. Why sleep deprivation makes us pale remains a mystery.

Another cause of pallor is anaemia, which is a decline in the number of red blood cells or their overall haemoglobin content. Anaemia has many causes, some of them very serious. If pallor persists for days and is accompanied by fatigue, go and see a doctor.

Goose bumps are another classic element of the fight-or-flight response, though not a very useful one. They are caused by the involuntary contraction of tiny muscles in the hair follicles called arrector pili muscles, which connect the base of the hair to the skin. When they contract – which is tiggered by both emotional arousal and cold – they hoist the hair aloft. This reflex is called piloerection, as in erection of a hair, or more descriptively horripilation, which is derived from the Latin word 'to bristle', which is also the root of the word 'horror'.

Horripilation is a vestigial reflex. It would have made our hairier ancestors look bigger and scarier, as when a cat bristles, and also would have made their fur a more effective insulation against the cold. Nowadays it doesn't achieve either. Some people can go goose-pimply at will, though how they consciously override their involuntary reflex is not known, and it is hardly a skill that any of us yearn for.

B.O. and smelly feet

As I worked on this book, I kept the title and contents a secret from all but my closest family and friends. Every now and then I'd tell somebody, 'You're in it.' They'd usually react with a mixture of pride and curiosity, but then I'd lie awake at night wondering what they would say (or do) when they found out I had written about their piles or crabs or strange beliefs about lip balm.

Fortunately, both for me and them, all of my friends and family have impeccable personal hygiene. So I don't have anyone to humiliate, even anonymously, about their malodorous armpits or feet. Except perhaps myself.

Everyone smells. Like it or not, body odour is a normal and unavoidable consequence of being human. That is because everybody produces skin secretions, and everybody's skin is colonised from head to toe with bacteria and other microorganisms that like to eat secretions and then fart out waste products. That is not to say that body odour is invariably unpleasant. Everybody has their own unique smell, some sweeter than others. Smell is also in the nose of the beholder; some people's body odour may smell awful to you but nice to me.

For that reason alone, I think it is time to stop using the term 'body odour' as a pejorative term. For that we can blame the ever-socially-responsible advertising industry, which in the 1920s hit on the idea that playing on people's insecurities, or even creating them, shifted product. The acronym B.O. first appeared in a deodorant advert in 1919; it cunningly did not reveal what B.O. stood for but urged women to perform the 'armhole odour test' to find out if they had it. In his 1936 novel

Keep the Aspidistra Flying, George Orwell satirically recounts how his anti-hero advertising copywriter Gordon Comstock invented the term Pedic Perspiration to exploit anxiety about sweaty feet. 'Once you knew what they stood for, you couldn't possibly see those letters "P.P." without a guilty tremor.'

Body odour is influenced by many factors but by far the most important is the action of microorganisms on the secretions of specialised glands, called apocrine glands, tucked inside hair follicles. These are modified sweat glands that, unlike the regular ones that produce mostly saltwater to cool us down, secrete a cloudy liquid mixture of oils, proteins, carbohydrates and steroids. This mixes with another oily secretion of the follicles, sebum, and leaks out onto the skin like a free milkshake fountain for hungry bacteria.

The regular (eccrine) sweat glands are distributed all over the body but the apocrine ones are concentrated in certain areas: the armpits, genitals, navel, ear canals, eyelids, nipples, nostrils and the area in front of the anus. Yes, they are definitely involved in sex.

Fresh apocrine sweat is odourless but when bacteria get to work on it they convert it into a pungent cocktail of organic waste molecules. These variously smell cheesy, oniony, floral, vinegary and rancid. They are not necessarily unpleasant, especially when combined with other human smells such as skin. Just as a fine wine may actually be improved by a hint of wet dog or cat pee, or a perfume by a waft of whale faeces extracted from ambergris, these ostensibly foul compounds can be oddly attractive. It is impossible to deny that a certain level of body odour can be really sexy. But there are limits. Failure to wash regularly – both skin and clothes – allows odours to build up to extremely pungent and intolerable levels.

Some people, by dint of their genes, the makeup of their skin microbiomes and their diets, get to that threshold faster. Men have more apocrine glands so tend to be ahead of that particular curve. But we all stink sooner or later.

Getting rid of bad body odour is as easy as soap and water. Washing gets rid of the bad-smelling compounds and flushes away at least some of the odour-producing bacteria. Underarm chemical warfare can help too. Antiperspirants bung up the apocrine glands for a while – there is no evidence that doing so is harmful – and deodorants mask the bad smells.

One question that often comes up in relation to body malodour is, can you tell if you have it? Or to put it more cruelly, why don't smelly people know they smell? The answer is that we can whiff ourselves to some extent, but like all bad smells that hang around like, er, a bad smell, we eventually become habituated to our own B.O. One trick for revealing the smelliness of one's own armpits is borrowed from the perfume industry. Before smelling your armpit, sniff some coffee beans. This resets the sense of smell and de-habituates it.

Habituation may also explain the mystery of how people in bygone days, when baths were an occasional luxury and laundry the thing you did in spring once it was warm enough to shed a few layers of clothing, could tolerate each other's odours, let alone get close enough to produce the next generation of smelly little monsters.

As Orwell predicted, smelly feet are just as much of a social stigma as stinky armpits. The causes of what is medically called bromodosis are essentially the same: bacteria chowing down on sweat. And, in the case of feet, dead skin. This extra menu item attracts a group of bacteria called *Brevibacteria*, which eat skin and excrete a colourless but definitely not odourless sulphurous gas called methanethiol. We will encounter this diabolical compound in more detail when I get on to flatulence, but suffice to say for now that it stinks to high heaven. Many cheeses that trade on their pungency emit clouds of the stuff, including the notoriously whiffy Limburger.

The answer, again, is simple: good hygiene and fresh air. I have a theory that the pandemic will have done wonders for our collective bromodosis problem, if not our armpits. Home workers are not obligated to wear shoes. Or take showers.

There is also a condition called pitted keratolysis that is (thankfully) mostly confined to the feet and brings an extra dimension to foot odour. You would not, repeat NOT, want it in your armpits. It is a bacterial infection which bores into the skin of the soles of the feet and gives them a pitted and spongy surface not unlike a crumpet or scotch pancake – or, for fans of exotic food, the spongy Ethiopian bread injera which I once saw described as looking and tasting like mouldy bandages. The bacteria responsible also emit sulphurous gases that I can confirm are the absolute pits. I had pitted keratolysis for years which I failed to deal with, thinking it was some form of athlete's foot. A bar of antibacterial soap and a scrubbing brush keep a lid on it, but my feet are still prone to straying into the Limburger zone.

I sincerely hope this act of self-shaming stands in my favour when my friends and family seek revenge.

3

Ear, Nose and Throat

Back in the day when people used to actually go to work, my route to and from *New Scientist* HQ took me past various venerable London medical institutions: Great Ormond Street Hospital, the Institute of Neurology, the British Medical Association, the National Hospital for Neurology and Neurosurgery and the Eastman Dental Institute. And then of course, a little further up the Gray's Inn Road, there was the Royal National Throat, Nose and Ear Hospital. I always regarded this as a bit of a medical backwater. Throats, noses and ears? Surely not the sharpest scalpels in the drawer.

As a result of writing this book, I have completely changed my mind and now hold ear, nose and throat doctors in the highest possible esteem. The lower half of the head is a magnificently intricate and wonderful part of the human body: a labyrinth of interconnected tunnels and chambers, tiny bones, complex surfaces, delicate muscles, vital organs of the immune system and even a beautifully engineered crumple zone.

Neurologists are often regarded as the glamorous heroes of medicine, but I think that another variety of head doctor deserve at least as much credit. So here's to the otorhinolaryngologists, the unsung heroes of one of the most amazing areas of the human body – the ears, nose and throat.

Earwax

As internet rabbit holes go, it is hard to beat earholes. Before writing this chapter, I spent more time than I care to admit watching YouTube videos of people having their earwax removed. Disgusting, yes. But very, very satisfying. It is amazing how much earwax one earhole can accumulate. The old expression 'you could grow potatoes in those ears' never seemed more apt.

Earwax is one of the more interesting secretions of the human body, though would not actually be a hospitable growth medium for potatoes. Technically called cerumen, it is a smelly and viscous mixture of fats, alcohols and cholesterol plus gubbins such as dead skin, dirt, sweat and small creatures. Some people are more prolific than others, but everybody produces it. And we make a lot of frankly pointless and actively harmful efforts to get rid of it.

Ear canals make wax for a reason. It is primarily a defence against insects, bacteria, fungi and other would-be invaders, which are repelled by the smell or become mired in the sticky wax. It also keeps the canal clean through a conveyor-belt mechanism whereby newly-secreted wax – from both sebaceous glands like the ones that are found all over the body and specialist ceruminous glands – flushes older wax outwards, aided by jaw movements. It also keeps the skin lining the canal moist and flexible.

There are two basic types of human earwax, wet and dry. Most people of African and European descent have the wet type, which is soft, moist and sticky and ranges from dark brown through bright orange to light yellow. Most people of East Asian and Native American descent have the dry type, which is flaky, crusty and grey. The difference is controlled by a single gene which is also involved in sweatiness; dry waxers have much fewer sweat glands and sweat a lot less than wet waxers. Why this gene variant persists is not known; it may be advantageous in certain climates. The earwax differences are a byproduct of this genetic change, as the ceruminous glands are actually modified sweat glands.

Ears are usually self-cleaning. But sometimes the rate of wax secretion exceeds removal and the ear canal becomes clogged. That can cause gradual hearing loss (often so gradual that we don't notice), earache, dizziness, itchiness and tinnitus (see page 141).

Various factors can accelerate the production of earwax or promote its accumulation to spud-worthy levels. Some people naturally make a lot of the stuff. Some have narrow or excessively hairy ear canals, which inhibit wax from dropping out. Older people produce harder wax. Being hot and sweaty promotes earwax secretion, which is why ears are sometimes prolifically waxy after a big night out or an intense bout of exercise.

At this point it is tempting to insert a cotton bud and rummage around, but this is not a good idea. It usually backfires, forcing the wax deeper into the ear like a ramrod cramming gunpowder into a muzzle. And if you do succeed, the glands compensate by upping their production.

The simplest way to get rid of compacted earwax is to put two or three drops of olive or almond oil into the ear canal to moisten and loosen the compacted plug and allow it to slide out under the influence of gravity. Back in the day, before we caught up with our European neighbours and realised that food was something to be enjoyed rather than endured, the only place in Britain where olive oil could be purchased was a pharmacy. Chemists still sell earwax-dissolving liquids, which do the same thing. If these fail, professional earwax removal may be required.

This used to be known as 'having your ears syringed',

because doctors would use a big metal syringe to squirt warm water into the ear and then suck it back out again. These days they use automated irrigators.

Ear candles, which are narrow fabric tubes soaked in wax that are inserted into the ear so they drip hot wax into it, do not work and can cause injuries. Most health authorities advise against them. As the US Food and Drug Administration advises, don't get burned. Exactly why anyone believes that a procedure that puts yet more wax into a clogged ear can unclog it is beyond me. Maybe they misheard.

Microsuction is perhaps the technique of last resort. The wax-removal professional peers into the ear with an instrument called an otoscope and uses tiny tools to scrape, tweeze and suck out the wax. Sometimes they film it and put it on YouTube. Which reminds me, I must go. I have some videos to watch . . .

Earache

The seventeenth-century physician and anatomist Jean Riolan the Younger clearly *wasn't* the sharpest scalpel in the drawer. Despite being the son of a renowned French anatomist (Jean Riolan the Elder) and a member of the Medical Faculty of Paris, he held some decidedly eccentric views about human biology. He disputed William Harvey's discoveries about the circulation of the blood, arguing that heartbeats were caused by the movement of the blood, not the other way round. He also believed that blood only returned to the heart twice or three times a day. He denied the existence of the recently discovered lymphatic system (see page 233). Nevertheless, in 1649 he made a discovery for which generations of hard-of-hearing children, and more recently fans of stop-motion animation, can be eternally grateful.

In typical Riolian fashion, he made it by accident after botching a routine procedure. While cleaning out a patient's ear canal with an ear spoon, he perforated their eardrum. The patient – who presumably was thought to be suffering from compacted earwax (see page 135) – reported an instant improvement in his hearing. The myringotomy had been invented.

Piercing of the eardrum is now routinely used to clear up glue ear, a common childhood condition in which the middle ear – an empty echo chamber between the eardrum and the delicate hearing apparatus of the inner ear – fills with fluid. The exact cause is unknown; it may be a malfunction of the Eustachian tube, which equalises pressure on either side of the eardrum. If the tube becomes blocked for some reason, air pressure in the middle ear drops, forcing fluid in from the surrounding tissue to make up the difference. Over time this thickens to a glue-like consistency and gums up one or both ear canals, frequently with serious repercussions for hearing. It often causes tinnitus (see page 141) and can hurt.

Glue ear is technically called otitis media with effusion, which is just a fancy way of saying infection of the middle ear with fluid accumulation. It is most prevalent in children, perhaps because they tend to have large and inflammation-prone pharyngeal tonsils, a.k.a. adenoids (see page 157), which can block the Eustachian tube. Adenoids and glue ear are common bedfellows and it is reasonable to assume that one leads to the other. However, no causal relation-ship has been firmly established, and in any case it cannot be the whole story. The pharyngeal tonsil shrinks during childhood, or is whipped out by a surgeon. Either way it has disappeared completely by adulthood. But adults can also get glue ear.

The condition usually resolves itself within three months, but chronic or recurrent cases require minor surgery as the hardness-of-hearing caused by glue ear can be a real handicap and interfere with a young child's language devel-opment. An ear, nose and throat surgeon will pierce the eardrum, which both allows the glue to ooze slowly out and prevents it from building up again. The perforation will naturally heal in a matter of weeks so is usually kept open using a small plastic eyelet called a tympanostomy tube, also called a transtympanic ventilation tube or, in plain English, a grommet. These are inserted into the hole in the eardrum under local or general anaesthetic. They stay in place for about a year then fall out, whereupon glue may start building up again, necessitating a replacement grommet.

Eardrums – which are thin membranes of the connective tissue collagen covered with skin, and are also called the tympanic membrane or myringa – can also be perforated by accident. The usual cause is a physical trauma such as ram-ming an ear spoon into the ear, or an infection of one or both of the chambers either side of it, the outer and middle ear. Sudden changes in pressure can also overstretch the eardrum and rupture it. Rapid ascent or descent in a plane, or diving too deep in water, can do this. So can the pressure wave from a very loud noise such as an explosion, or even just blowing your nose too hard. Perforated eardrums hurt and can cause hearing loss, but they usually heal by themselves. If not, the same sort of surgeon who perforates eardrums for a living can also un-perforate them.

Pressure changes can also cause eardrums to hurt without stretching them to destruction. The solution is to swallow or chew, which opens the Eustachian tube and equalises the pressure. This can also happen spontaneously; this is what causes the ears to 'pop', often followed by sudden clarity in hearing, when gradually changing altitude.

Infections of the outer ear and middle ear – called otitis externa and otitis media – are also common causes of ear pain. Otitis externa is sometimes called 'swimmer's ear' because getting water in the ear – where it often remains for hours, sloshing about in an annoying way like you've got an entire swimming pool in there – can soften the skin and make it susceptible to infection. Lie on your side and let gravity work its magic. Ear plugs or a swimming cap pulled over the ears should stop water getting in in the first place. You can also buy ear drops that lubricate the ear canal and help water to trickle back out. Bad ear infections can cause pain, hearing loss, tinnitus and the leakage of foul-smelling pus from the ears, but are easily cleared up with medications from the chemist or a doctor.

Infections of the inner ear – called otitis interna or labyrinthitis – are much more unpleasant. They interfere with hearing and with the vestibular system which senses the position of the head, leading to sickening vertigo, often severe enough to cause vomiting. Labyrinthitis can come on suddenly and last for several debilitating weeks. Very similar symptoms are also caused by vestibular neuritis, inflammation of the nerve in the inner ear that communicates with the brain. Both require treatment.

Anyway, back to grommets. They are also used to help people who, perhaps because of an inherited defect in their Eustachian tubes, struggle to equalise pressure in the ear and so get really painful earache on aeroplanes.

The undeniably comical word 'grommet' is forever associated with glue ear (also undeniably comical), but it is actually a venerable Old French nautical word for a circle of rope. Sadly, *gromette* is now obsolete and the French have to make do with the distinctly uncomical *oeillet*.

The word 'grommet' – which is not really a medical term but a general one for a ring or washer inserted into a sheet of material – was also the inspiration for the name of the dog in Nick Park's brilliant *Wallace & Gromit* animation series, though sadly this has nothing to do with glue ear. According to the official Wallace and Gromit website, Park's older brother was an electrician who often talked about grommets; Park thought it would make a brilliant name for a cartoon animal. Interestingly, dogs also get glue ear. Grommet, Gromit?

Tinnitus and earworms

Sometimes, usually when I'm about to get into the shower, one of the most annoying songs ever pops into my head and takes up residence there. I can't dislodge it and the more I try, the more annoying it gets. I can hear every detail, with painful clarity. What have I done to deserve this torture? 'We Built This City (on Rock and Roll)' by Starship was terrible when it first came out in 1985, and it hasn't improved with age.

But look on the bright side: at least it drowns out the ringing in my ears.

Most people at some point in their lives experience a persistent phantom sound. Earworms and tinnitus are extremely common and very varied but they do share one feature: they are extraordinarily, infuriatingly annoying.

They also mostly have nothing to do with actual sound: both are largely a product of your brain, not your ears. That is obviously true of earworms but also of tinnitus, which is medically defined as being able to hear sound when none is actually present.

The word comes from the Latin *tinnio*, 'to ring or jingle', and the classic manifestation is a bell-like ringing. But almost every conceivable annoying noise has been reported, from pure tones through static, screeching, humming, sizzling, grating, whistling, hissing, clicking, roaring, beeping, buzzing, cicada-like chirping and even sounds resembling singing or speech. Many people experience two or more noises, often simultaneously, and it is possible to have different ones 'in' your left and right ears. The noises can come and go or be constant, and the volume varies from barely noticeable to deafening. Tinnitus torments roughly one in six people during their lives.

Most just learn to live with it; in parts of India it is actually considered a blessing, as it means the gods are speaking to you directly. But around a quarter of people end up seeking medical help because the noise drives them up the wall, keeps them awake at night or interferes with their concentration.

Tinnitus is not a condition in itself but a symptom of some underlying cause, almost always quite trivial. Around 90 per cent of people with it have some degree of hearing loss, sometimes simply due to an ear infection or build-up of earwax (see page 135). It can also be due to glitches in the brain pathways that process sound.

During the Covid-19 pandemic, tinnitus emerged as one of the more unusual and inexplicable symptoms of the disease. People who already had tinnitus often reported that it worsened when they were ill, and some people 'caught' tinnitus along with Covid-19. Tinnitus has also been reported as a symptom of the lingering after-effects of the virus, known as long Covid.

Another common cause is damage to the hairs on auditory cells. That is why exposure to loud noises, such as a rock concert or explosion, can produce a temporary ringing in the ears: they inflict temporary damage on auditory hairs. If the damage is permanent and your hearing is partially lost, getting a hearing aid can solve both problems. Some people find that adding genuine background noise such as music, a fan or a white-noise generator masks the tinnitus.

Despite tinnitus being defined as phantom noise, it can sometimes be real, caused by turbulent blood-flow in veins or arteries in the head or problems with the joint connecting the jawbone to the skull. A handful of rare causes are serious, including diabetes and multiple sclerosis. So it is worth getting tinnitus checked out, especially if it is getting worse.

If earwax removal, a hearing aid or background noise doesn't work, your options are limited. There are no drugs or medical devices that are approved for tinnitus, though an experimental therapy that feeds sound into the ears while simultaneously stimulating the tongue with a weak electrical current for an hour a day has produced some encouraging results. But while we wait for that device to be approved, cognitive behavioural therapy and counselling can help. There's also 'tinnitus retraining therapy', which basically means learning to ignore the noise.

Another inner sound you basically have to learn to ignore is the earworm. These are even more common than tinnitus. One study done in Finland in 2008 found that 90 per cent of people experience them at least weekly and a third of people daily.[20]

The word is of German origin – *Ohrwurm* means 'earwig', which were commonly believed to crawl into people's ears, burrow into their brains and lay their eggs there (they don't). Germans apparently started calling stuck-in-your-head songs *Ohrwurms* in the 1950s and the term crept into English in the 1980s.

Earworms are known in neuroscience circles as involuntary musical imagery and are a form of 'spontaneous cognition', which is an umbrella term for thoughts, emotions and memories that come to mind without being invoked deliberately or triggered by an external stimulus. Daydreaming and mind-wandering are a form of spontaneous cognition, and they turn out to be what our brains are doing most of the time.

This spontaneous cognition is thought to be important for processing past events and planning future ones, though what if any part earworms play in that is not known.

Songs that worm their way in are typically catchy, upbeat pop tunes with lyrics. Lady Gaga is a serial offender; in a recent survey to find the most common earworms she had the number one hit with 'Bad Romance' and two other songs, 'Alejandro' and 'Poker Face', in the top ten. Appropriately,

'Can't Get You Out of my Head' by Kylie Minogue came in at number two.

Catchy, upbeat pop songs are arguably the most annoying musical genre, which is probably why earworms tend to be so irritating. If you are being tormented by one, a tried and tested way to purge it is to listen to the actual song. So I am going to have to bite the bullet: 'We built this city . . . we built this city on rock 'n' roll, built this city . . .'

Nosebleeds

One of the more creative entries in the lexicon of football commentary clichés is the nosebleed. This is when a defensive player finds him or herself in the opposition penalty box with the ball at their feet and the goal at their mercy, only to shank it over the bar. 'Oof, (s)he's had a nosebleed,' the commentator will inevitably scoff. In other words, he or she ventured far too high up the pitch and the altitude got to them.

Nosebleeds can be triggered by altitude, but it has nothing to do with pressure. The air is usually dryer up there, which can cause the inside of the nose to desiccate, crack and bleed.

There usually isn't much more to nosebleeds than that. The majority of what doctors call an epistaxis are anterior nosebleeds, which means that the blood is leaking from the wall of the septum, the piece of soft tissue separating the nostrils. The skin there is delicate, rich in blood vessels, and easily broken. Cold, dry air is a common cause, as are nose-picking and vigorous nose-blowing.

The other sort of bleed, the posterior nosebleed, comes from the blood vessels higher up in the nasal cavity. They can also be caused by cold, nose-blowing and fingernails, though it is an adventurous nose-picker who goes that far in. Posterior nosebleeds tend to be heavier and involve blood coming from both nostrils rather than one. Blood can also trickle down the back of the throat.

Nosebleeds in general are more common in children, whose nasal vasculature is still developing and may be extra-delicate, and also elderly people with aged and papery skin and low levels of clot-promoting platelets in their blood, a condition commonly called thin blood (medics, unsurprisingly, have a posher-sounding name for it, thrombocytopenia, which means 'platelet poverty'). Hormonal changes during pregnancy can also thin the blood, and nosebleeds are a common inconvenience for pregnant women.

A few underlying conditions make nosebleeds more likely, such as high blood pressure, hardening of the arteries and blood-clotting disorders. Anticoagulants such as warfarin list nosebleeds as a possible side effect, and you are advised to contact a doctor if one occurs while you're taking this medication.

When a nosebleed strikes, standard medical advice is to sit or stand upright to reduce the blood pressure in the nasal veins, pinch the soft part of the nose just above the nostrils for fifteen minutes, lean forward a bit to stop the blood from flowing down your throat, and put an ice pack on the bridge of the nose. If you can do all those at once, you're well on the way back to rude health. Avoid the temptation to stuff a plug of toilet paper up the offending nostril as it can make the injury worse and become stuck to the coagulating blood, risking a repeat performance when it is pulled out.

If the nosebleed doesn't stop after fifteen minutes or seems excessively heavy it is a good idea to see a doctor – though by the time you actually see one you may have bled out. They have magic sticks called styptic pencils that can be applied to the location of the bleeding and stop it instantly. The active ingredient is anhydrous aluminium sulphate, which is very dry and astringent and causes blood vessels to clench up. They are available to buy and also used on shaving cuts (see page 316).

Nosebleeds occasionally happen during sleep, and are not discovered until awakening in a pool (okay, splotch) of blood. Maybe they are caused by dreams about finding yourself in the opposition penalty box with the ball at your feet and the goal at your mercy . . .

Sinusitis

You've got holes in your head, and sometimes they fill with snot. But don't worry – you can always flush them out with salty water. My father-in-law is a master of this, a result of years of practice. He suffers from chronic sinusitis and can often be seen with a decongestant stick in one or other nostril, or sometimes both. The double-nostril look is known as 'the walrus' and is a sure-fire warning that some violent snorting is on the horizon.

Sinusitis is inflammation of the paranasal sinuses, a cluster of eight air-filled cavities in the front of the skull which connect to the nasal passage. There are four pairs in a circle around the centre of the face. Their volume can add up to 60 millilitres, which is about the same as a double whisky.

They are often just referred to as 'sinuses' but that is an anatomy school error; a sinus is a cavity in any organ. They are found all over the body, from the brain to the anus. That is not an area where you want to have sinusitis.

The function of the parasinuses has been the topic of much anatomical debate, but they mainly appear to heat and moisten inhaled air before it descends to the lungs. They also produce mucus and feed it into the nostrils, help to amplify speech, and stop your head from being too heavy. And they are good in an emergency, acting as a crumple zone to minimise serious damage from being hit in the face.

They are also annoyingly prone to getting inflamed. Infections, allergies and air pollution can all cause the lining of the parasinuses to swell up, which can inflict pain and discomfort in and around the face. The swelling can also block the small orifices, called ostia, which link them to the nasal cavity and thus prevent the sinuses from draining properly. The consequent build-up of mucus just adds to the discomfort.

Sinusitis is most often caused by an infection, usually by the same motley crew of viruses that cause the common cold (see page 224). Around 2 per cent of colds and flu progress to sinusitis.

In fact, most colds feature a mild secondary infection of the paranasal sinuses, often set up by vigorous nose-blowing. Back in the year 2000, a team of doctors recruited four people with colds and measured the pressure they created inside their noses when they blew them. They measured thirty-five nose-blows in total, and found that the average pressure wave was about ten times as much as generated by a sneeze. This, they concluded, was enough to propel virus-laden snot from the nose into the parasinuses.

Once the infection sets in, it can be hard to shift. A bout usually lasts at least two weeks and can go on for months. As well as pain and congestion it can lead to a dulled sense of smell, headaches, thick green snot, fever, toothache (one pair of parasinuses is located close to the upper jaw) and bad breath.

The answer is rest, painkillers and plenty of fluids, which has been shown to loosen the snot a little. Volatile oils such as eucalyptus can achieve similar results by irritating the lining of the parasinuses and increasing the flow of fresh, watery mucus. Many over-the-counter decongestants contain a drug called xylometazoline, which causes blood vessels to constrict and so reduces swelling. But overuse of this drug can induce tolerance, which just exacerbates the problem. When the drug is stopped the congestion comes back with a vengeance, a condition called rhinitis medicamentosa or rebound congestion.

Tolerance is not a problem for the old-fashioned home remedy favoured by my father-in-law. The procedure goes like this: boil a pint of water and dissolve a teaspoon of salt and a teaspoon of bicarbonate of soda into it. Wash your hands thoroughly. When the solution has cooled enough, pour some into the palm of your cupped hand, lift it to the nose, block one nostril and inhale vigorously. Repeat until the congestion eases. Or you cannot tolerate any more.

Mouth ulcers

When I was a teenager, I was prone to getting mouth ulcers, which my mum always said was a sure sign that I was 'a bit run down'. It made intuitive sense; I was burning the candle at both ends and ate a diet that would give a modern nutritionist heartburn. If she was begging me to be more sensible, it didn't work. My own teenage son is now prone to mouth ulcers, which we also invariably attribute to him being a bit run down.

We'll get to the 'run down' thing in due course. Mouth ulcers – which usually appear on the insides of the cheeks or lips, and sometimes under or on the underside of the tongue – are very common. Around 70 per cent of people in western countries get one at some point in their lives and 20 per cent are plagued by recurrent outbreaks.

There are two basic types of mouth ulcer. They can be caused by an injury, such as biting the inside of a cheek, a slip of the toothbrush, abrasion by a broken tooth or a burn from hot food or drink. These traumatic ulcers are simply wounds, and heal naturally in a few days.

The other type – the ones associated with run-downness – usually strike out of the blue though are also associated with menstruation. The technical name of the condition is aphthous stomatitis, which translates as 'ulcerous inflammation of the mouth and lips'. They are also called canker sores.

An ulcer is any breach in the skin where the top layer has been stripped away and the underlying tissue is necrotic, which means dying or dead. In the case of mouth ulcers, the top layer is the mucosal surface of the mouth or tongue. Exactly why it breaks down is not clear. Mouth ulcers are not caused by an infection and are not contagious, though can become infected.

The ulcers themselves are irregular patches of whitish broken skin, often with a red rim. They are usually no more than a few millimetres across but can occur in clusters called 'crops'. People who are ulcer-prone grow a new crop every few months. They can be sore, but generally heal on their own after a few days. There are various creams, lotions and mouthwashes that ease the irritation and promote healing.

Some people have it really bad. Major aphthous ulceration produces large, deep and raw ulcers that can take weeks to heal, often leaving a scar. Even worse is herpetiform recurrent aphthous stomatitis, which is characterised by mass outbreaks of tiny ulcers that can join forces to make one really big and very painful one. Herpetiform means 'resembling herpes', which reflects a long-held but erroneous medical belief that ulcers are herpes, or cold sores (see page 250). Like the other forms of aphthous stomatitis, the herpetiform one is not caused by any virus, let alone the herpes one, and is not contagious.

The actual cause of mouth ulcers is not known. They run in families and may be an autoimmune condition, meaning that the body mistakenly launches an immune attack on its own tissues.

There are some well-established triggers in people who have recurrent ulcers. One is stress; another is iron or vitamin B12 deficiency. Both might reasonably also be seen as 'being a bit run down', which is just a folk name for fatigue. But fatigue itself does not seem to be a risk factor.

Another possible trigger is a common ingredient of toothpaste and mouthwash, sodium lauryl sulphate, which is basically a type of mouth soap. Some people find that avoiding it reduces their attacks of ulcers, but doing so is easier said than done; it is both cheap and very effective and an almost ubiquitous ingredient of oral hygiene products. When the US healthcare company Johnson & Johnson discontinued a sodium lauryl sulphate-free toothpaste in 2014, tubes of it started changing hands on the internet for ten times the retail price. The company quickly dis-discontinued it.

Mouth ulcers are not always nothing much to worry about. Some forms of oral cancer start life looking very similar to an outbreak of aphthous stomatitis. Ulcers that do not go away in three weeks are worth getting checked out.

Many other diseases also cause mouth ulcers. One is hand, foot and mouth disease (not to be confused with foot and mouth disease of cattle and sheep), which is one of those common and largely harmless infections of childhood. It makes you feel a bit under the weather for a couple of days then erupts into ulcers inside the mouth and (you guessed it) on the hands and feet. It is caused by a group of different viruses and generally goes away, though sometimes people's fingernails and toenails fall off a month or so after recovering from it.

I'm feeling a bit run down after all of this. Luckily for me, mouth ulcers become less common as we age, and I haven't had one for years. Early night for me, again . . .

Sore tongue

According to traditional Chinese medicine, the tongue is a window on the soul. Well, the internal organs anyway. Practitioners place great faith in being able to diagnose diseases by inspecting the colour and texture of a patient's tongue. A pale tongue with red spots, a thin white coating and teeth marks around the edge is diagnostic of Qi deficiency, for example, which manifests as low energy, sweatiness and bruising. Someone with Yin deficiency – which causes emaciation, insomnia and thin urine – will have a red, cracked tongue. Why the doctor cannot just ask the patient about their symptoms I do not know.

Tongue diagnosis has been around for about 2,000 years – its principles are spelled out in a medical treatise called the *Esoteric Scripture of the Yellow Emperor*, thought to have been written during the Han dynasty – but cannot be accused of failing to move with the times. Doctors in China now use it to diagnose various stages of Covid-19.[21]

I won't say anything about the veracity of the TCM tongue fetish except to paraphrase the always-quotable football manager Ron Atkinson: I never comment on alternative medicine and I'm not going to break the habit of a lifetime for that rubbish (Atkinson was asked for his thoughts about a referee, and used the word 'prat').

Western medicine also concerns itself with irregularities of the tongue, and a doctor will often ask their patient to stick it out so they can have a butcher's. Some tongue problems are definitely indicative of underlying conditions. A sore, red tongue can be a symptom of all sorts of nutrient deficiencies, for example. But on the whole, what happens on the tongue stays on the tongue.

Aside from a few rare exceptions – furrows can be a symptom of syphilis and a thick white fur on the side of the tongue, called hairy leukoplakia, is caused by a virus and can be a sign of immune deficiency – tongue disorders are not regarded as signs of underlying conditions.

Broadly, there are two things that can go wrong with tongues. They can become red and sore (called glossitis, from *glóssa*, the Greek for 'tongue', as in glossolalia), or develop white patches. Or both.

One fairly common form of glossitis is the brilliantly named geographical tongue, so-called because of irregular red patches on the upper surface that resemble the outlines of land masses on a map. The cause is erosion of the skin of the tongue, for no apparent reason. It usually doesn't hurt. Another condition with a fantastically descriptive name is strawberry tongue, in which the tongue swells and reddens, making the white taste buds stand out like seeds on a strawberry. Sometimes the taste buds also turn red, which is known as raspberry tongue. Both are a classic early symptom of scarlet fever (see page 244).

On the white side, mouth ulcers (see page 150), oral thrush (see page 256) and the skin condition called lichen planus (see page 101) are major causes. There's also non-hairy leukoplakia, which, as its name suggests, is characterised by flat white plaques on the tongue. The plaques can't be scraped away. The cause is unknown but it is worth keeping an eye as the plaques are considered a pre-cancerous lesion, meaning they very occasionally progress to cancer.

All too often, however, a white fur on the tongue is simply a sign of poor oral hygiene. A Chinese doctor would diagnose you with Yang deficiency, but a toothbrush or tongue scraper and some elbow grease should see the back of it quickly enough.

Tonsillitis

When I was a kid, I always wanted to have my tonsils out. Not because I was a chronic sufferer of tonsillitis but because there was a rumour that if you asked the doctor nicely, he (doctors were always he in those days) would give you them in a jar to take home. Unfortunately, I never found out whether or not this was true, though years later it emerged that Prince Charles had his tonsils out as a child and was given them in a jar of formaldehyde which he carried around with him at all times. So it must have been true. Believe me, I would have done the same.

Back in those days there was also a great deal of confusion about what tonsils actually were. Loads of kids had them removed, apparently with no ill effect, so what were they for? The playground consensus was that they must be useless left-overs a bit like appendices, which were also being whipped out of kids at my school at an alarming rate (and, yes, you could keep those in a jar too).

The tonsils that were being separated from their owners were actually called the palatine tonsils, a pair of pink and squishy organs located at the back of the throat. Open your mouth wide and look in the mirror; unless you have been tonsillectomied, the palatine tonsils are those large-ish purplish blobs to the left and right of the dangly thing that is often mistaken for the epiglottis but is actually called the uvula. Locating the palatine tonsils has become something of a talking point in the age of Covid-19, as the self-administered test requires us to rub a swab on them before shoving it up the nose.

The palatine tonsils are part of a ring of six tonsils collectively called Waldeyer's lymphatic ring, which encircles the entrance to the windpipe and oesophagus and carries out immune surveillance of food, drink and air entering the body. They are the first line of defence against pathogens entering the lungs and digestive tract. The ring is named after its discoverer, German anatomist Heinrich Wilhelm Gottfried von Waldeyer-Hartz, who incidentally also coined the word 'chromosome'.

The full membership of the lymphatic ring is – starting at twelve o'clock – the pharyngeal tonsil (of which more later), two tubal tonsils, two palatine tonsils, and the lingual tonsil. This latter tonsil is anchored at the root of the tongue, hence its name.

All six tonsils are rich in immune cells including antibody-producing B-cells and T-cells, which among other things kill cells infected with viruses. Their surfaces are coated with another type of immune cell, the M-cell, which detects pathogens and alerts the B- and T-cells. If a pathogen enters the throat area, the tonsils make it their business to know about it and then kick the immune system into action.

Unfortunately, being on the frontline is dangerous and tonsils often get infected themselves. In the case of the palatine tonsils this is called tonsillitis, which causes them to become painfully swollen. It can come on rapidly and make it hard to swallow, both because the tonsils are enlarged and because it really hurts.

Tonsillitis is a leading cause of sore throats, though by no means the only one (see page 160). It is mostly caused by viruses such as those that cause flu and the common cold, but can also be bacterial. The viral disease infectious mononucleosis, or glandular fever, often causes nasty tonsilitis (see page 249). So does the bacterial disease streptococcal pharyngitis, commonly known as strep throat, which can spread from the pharynx to the tonsils.

Sometimes the red and swollen tonsils are embellished with small white blobs, which are sacs of pus – the remains of white blood cells that have made the ultimate sacrifice. Their rotting corpses can also make breath smell awful.

Bad cases of tonsillitis can make us feel absolutely lousy, like a bout of flu. Fever, cough, headache, earache, nausea and loss of voice are not uncommon. The lymph nodes in the neck can also become swollen and painful – they are immune organs not unlike the tonsils and will be working hard to fight the infection. The infection can spread to the other tonsils, especially the lingual tonsil at the base of the throat. The pharyngeal tonsil on the roof of the mouth can get infected too. An infected and swollen pharyngeal tonsil is called an adenoid (or adenoids, even though there is only one of them).

Adenoids are another common childhood problem. Due to infections or allergies, the tonsil can swell to the size of a ping-pong ball and obstruct breathing, leading to an annoyingly whiny, nasally voice. Adenoids are also associated with frequent ear infections and glue ear (see page 138). The solution: chop them off (not the ears). Adenoidectomy is one of the most common surgeries performed on children. It generally solves the glue ear problem and appears to have no ill-effect in the long term, perhaps because the pharyngeal tonsil is mostly active in early childhood and begins to shrink after about the age of seven. By adulthood it has dwindled to almost nothing.

There's not much that can be done for a bout of tonsillitis except to rest, take painkillers, gargle with warm salt water and/or soluble aspirin and sip cold drinks to soothe the pain. Antiseptic and anaesthetic throat sprays will also help. The infection usually clears up in a few days.

Children are at greater risk from tonsillitis, in part because their tonsils are bigger. Tonsils grow throughout childhood and peak at puberty then decline. If a child has multiple bouts of tonsillitis, the recommended course of action is to surgically remove them.

Tonsillectomy is a frequent source of controversy. It definitely reduces the incidence of palatine tonsillitis – you can't get an infection in an organ that is in a jar of formaldehyde – but some studies find that it does not reduce the overall number of acute sore throats, perhaps because there are four other tonsils for viruses and bacteria to attack. Other studies find that doctors are too quick to reach for the scalpel, with seven out of eight children who are tonsillectomied not reaching the agreed threshold – seven or more bouts of tonsillitis in a year, five or more bouts in each of the past two years or three or more in the past three. Chopping off tonsils also costs the health service a lot of money, and surgery has risks.

In 1930s Britain, tonsillectomy was routine, with more than half of children being deprived of their tonsils whether they needed them or not. That had more to do with doctors being paid per tonsillectomy than any real medical benefit. After the Second World War, a link was established between tonsillectomy and a form of polio, and the popularity of tonsillectomy dropped. But in 1964 it rose again after an unlikely celebrity endorsement. In June of that year, the Beatles were about to embark on their first ever world tour. Doing a photoshoot for the *Saturday Evening Post*, Ringo Starr – the drummer – fell ill with tonsillitis and was taken to hospital with a raging fever. Ringo's tonsils then became a national story as the Fab Three reluctantly agreed to go on tour without him; a session drummer was hastily recruited and given a mop-top haircut. Ringo had been in the band for less than two years after the dismissal of the original drummer, Pete Best, and the band did not want rumours to circulate that they had sacked Ringo too. So the publicist sent a photographer to the hospital to make sure that Ringo and his tonsils stayed in the news. He (and they) made a rapid recovery and rejoined the band in Australia a week later; in December Ringo's tonsils were back in the news after he had them removed.

By the 1970s – when I was at junior school – tonsillectomies were doing a roaring trade. But they fell out of fashion again when it became clear that the cash-strapped NHS was squandering millions on unnecessary operations, mostly for the worried well.

Nevertheless, the NHS still performs thousands of tonsillectomies. Every year about 2.5 children per 1,000 have their tonsils out. Sometimes the adenoids come out at the same time, in a procedure called an adenotonsillectomy.

As for the risks of living without palatine tonsils, there do not appear to be any. The immune system does not seem to miss them at all, which is odd – why bother to have them in the first place? You might as well chop them out and keep them in a jar by the door.

Sore throat

Infected tonsils are not the only thing that can make it feel like you are swallowing a mixture of gravel and broken glass. Other parts of the throat are also susceptible to viruses and bacteria. Sore throats are very common, often as a symptom of a wider disease such as a cold (see page 228) or infectious mononucleosis (glandular fever, see page 248), but sometimes on their own.

The pharynx, a fancy name for the back of the throat, is the usual site of the problem. But the deeper-lying larynx or voice box also catches a cold from time to time. For some obscure reason these infections are called pharyngitis and laryngitis when common sense would suggest pharynx- and larynxitis. But whoever accused medical terminology of common sense?

The infectious agent is usually a virus but bacteria also get in on the act. About a third of sore throats are caused by a group of closely related bacteria in the genus *Streptococcus*, which normally live harmlessly on the skin and inside the mouth but can attack the pharynx and cause it to swell painfully. This streptococcal pharyngitis – widely known as strep throat – is essentially impetigo of the back of the throat, though it doesn't produce cornflake-like crusts (see page 78).

Laryngitis also causes a sore throat but has the added bonus of making the voice sound hoarse, croaky or totally inaudible. A lost voice doesn't necessarily mean an infected larynx. Excess mucus, or phlegm, can clog it up, and excessive shouting can make it swell up.

The expression 'frog in your throat' was coined in the 1890s by a patent medicine company called Taylor Bros to advertise a throat sweet that it claimed was 'the greatest cough and throat lozenge on earth'. It chose a frog because of its croakiness, presumably. And maybe because the lozenge would cause users to hoik up something green and slimy. The expression is uniquely English, though other languages also pin the blame on animals. Italians say they have a 'toad in the throat'; the French go for a cat. Many Slavic languages say, 'I have a dumpling in my throat,' and Greeks say 'razor blades'.

Medicated lozenges are still widely used to soothe sore throats, but suckers beware: the NHS says that 'there isn't much scientific evidence to suggest they help'. It recommends water instead: gargle with warm, salty water, drink lots of cold water (don't mix up the glasses!), put out bowls of water at home to keep the air moist, and suck ice cubes. Painkillers can help too. Sore throats usually go away, and lost voices return, in a few days.

Coughs

Take a deep breath. Along with about half a litre of air, you have just breathed in a cocktail of dust, soot, droplets, pollutants, pollen, viruses, bacteria and fungal spores. It's enough to make anyone splutter. No wonder coughs are the single most common reason why people go to see their doctor.

And visits to the doctor are just the tip of the iceberg. Most people don't bother with an appointment, but head for the chemist instead. In the US, sales of cough remedies total several billion dollars a year. Which is a large proportion of several billion dollars down the drain as most of them don't do anything.

Everybody gets a cough from time to time. Coughing is a frequent symptom of the common cold (see page 222) and other respiratory tract infections, but can also occur on its own without sniffles and sneezes. The final lingering symptom of a cold is often a cough.

The coincidence of colds and coughs is no coincidence at all. The causes are often the same. Most acute coughs are upper respiratory tract infections – usually abbreviated to URTIs – with the same cast of characters that cause the common cold. When doctors in Australia swabbed the airways of more than 800 children with coughs to discover what was ailing them, they found an absolute menagerie of viruses and bacteria. More than 90 per cent of the kids were infected with at least one, and most had several. They had rhinoviruses, coronaviruses, influenza and parainfluenza viruses, respiratory syncytial viruses and metapneumoviruses, plus bacteria known to cause pneumonia, catarrh and bacterial flu.

We can of course now add a new virus to that list: SARS-CoV-2. One of the symptoms of the virus (but by no means the only one) is a new and persistent cough. Unlike the common coronaviruses, the new one can be deadly, largely because it can penetrate deep into the lungs and cause pneumonia, which is much more serious than an URTI. The pandemic has turned niggly coughs from something we used to grin and bear into a source of great anxiety.

Infectious coughs are usually triggered by the immune response rather than the infectious agent itself. Inflammation irritates the airways and triggers the cough reflex in a bid to expel the irritant. If the immune response is also generating mucus and phlegm, these can be expelled – or expectorated – in projectile quantities. This is what is known as a wet or productive cough. If there is no phlegm the cough is dry and tickly instead.

Coughs can also be triggered by physical irritants such as smoke and dust particles and chemical irritants such as acids. One of the most potent cough-inducing chemicals is capsaicin, the hot ingredient in chillies. Frying chillies in a wok is a very effective way of driving my wife out of the kitchen – for reasons unknown, women are more sensitive than men to tussigenic agents, the posh name for things that make us cough (*tussis* is Latin for 'cough'). But even capsaicin has nothing on resiniferatoxin, the most potent tussigen ever discovered. It is a natural insecticide produced by a succulent plant growing in the Atlas Mountains. It is a thousand times hotter than pure capsaicin but the toughest chilli heads wouldn't want to fry it up; even tiny quantities can burn the skin, mouth and airways and the fatal ingested dose for a human is estimated to be less than 2 grams. It and capsaicin are often used in coughing experiments on humans and lab guinea pigs, which in the case of coughing usually *are* guinea pigs as they have a very similar cough reflex to humans.

A cough happens in instalments. Specialist receptors in the airways send signals to a region of the brainstem called the cough centre, which initiates and coordinates a sequence of movements ending in the violent expulsion of air.

First, there is a sharp inhalation of breath. Once the lungs are full, the glottis closes to seal off the windpipe. The abdominal muscles then squeeze violently to force air out of the lungs and up to the closed glottis. Under intense pressure the glottis reopens and the air rushes out, which causes the characteristic barking sound and hopefully expels whatever it was that needed to be coughed up. Coughed air can travel at up to 18 kilometres an hour.

More often than not, the cough is only partially successful and the reflex recurs, sometimes several times a minute.

Coughs can be so violent that they wreak havoc elsewhere in the body. Really bad coughing fits can cause people to faint, vomit, poo and pee themselves, crack ribs, develop hernias, damage pelvic floor muscles and suffer minor haemorrhages in the eye. Coughs can also interfere with sleep, both of the person hacking away all night and anyone they share a house with.

Acute coughs caused by infections can sometimes linger for weeks, months or years, long after the infection itself has cleared up. Why this chronic cough develops is not known; one possibility is low-level damage to the airways that makes us more sensitive to other cough triggers. Chronic coughs are also triggered by many other things, the most common being asthma and something called 'post-nasal drip syndrome'. This is when excess mucus accumulates in the back of the nose and drips into the larynx where it irritates the cough receptors. Allergies and infections of the nose and sinuses can cause post-nasal dripping. So can acid reflux, when stomach acid escapes and rises up the oesophagus (see page 187). Acid reflux often turns out to be the underlying cause of otherwise-mysterious chronic coughs.

Regardless of the cause, coughs are a great source of medical misery. There is no shortage of over-the-counter cough mixtures available: expectorants to loosen phlegm, suppressors for dry coughs and demulcents to soothe a tickly throat. Chest rubs are very popular too. Problem is, there is little evidence that any of them work. A systematic review of over-the-counter cough medications found no good evidence for or against the effectiveness of any of them, and lots of instances of side effects such as nausea, headaches and drowsiness.[22] In a rare instance of folk wisdom not being hokum, the best of a bad bunch was honey. I will spare you the obvious pun about not coughing up. In any case, coughs happen for a reason and suppressing them is not necessarily a good idea. Get it off your chest.

Sneezing fits

Back in my undergraduate days, one of my flatmates and I discovered that we shared a strange and unusual affliction. Thinking about sex – a fairly common distraction among men in their early twenties, especially ones studying science at a university with a male to female ratio of about seven to one – made us both sneeze. I don't remember how we found that out but I do remember that once we did, whenever one of us sneezed we would say, 'I wasn't.' (I sometimes was. He *always* was.)

The sex sneeze is a real thing, for reasons we will get into. But it is not the usual cause of sneezing. What is technically called the sternutatory reflex mostly happens in response to something tickling the lining of the nose, such as pollen or noxious chemicals. This triggers a response designed to get rid of whatever is doing the tickling: deep breath, closure of the glottis, lifting of the tongue to partially close the oral cavity and open the nasal one, violent contractions of the chest and abdominal muscles to create high pressure in the trachea, pursing of the lips to further close the mouth, and a sudden re-opening of the glottis allowing a violent expulsion of air. This is almost exactly the same sequence as a cough (see page 164), except that the air is mostly forced out of the nose rather than the mouth. Like coughing, it is coordinated by a dedicated area of the brainstem, the sneezing centre.

The classic 'achoo!' sound has been explained as a natural product of the sneezing action. The preparatory inhalation creates the 'a' (or 'a-a-a-a' in the build-up to a really major sneeze) and then rapid exhalation with the tongue on the roof of the mouth and the lips pursed naturally generates a 'choo'. But in fact sneeze sounds are significantly shaped by language and culture, though all are variations on a theme. French speakers go '*atchoum*', Japanese '*hakashun*', Polish '*a-psik*' and Vietnamese '*hat-xi*'. Deaf people often sneeze almost silently. When you go 'achoo', you are half-sneezing, half-speaking.

Of all the methods of expulsion invented by the human body, the sneeze is the most explosive. Droplets have been clocked travelling at 6 metres per second, or 21.6 kilometres an hour, which beats coughing by about 1 metre per second.

The sneezing action is a set of coordinated, finely tuned movements involving muscles in the abdomen, windpipe, throat and eyelids. It is common knowledge that the eyes close to prevent eyeballs from popping out of their sockets, and that sneezing with your eyes open is impossible. Both are myths. The eyes do usually close, but why is a mystery.

Sneezes are not in themselves dangerous, though cases of whiplash have been recorded. But they are often a symptom of illness, which is why in many cultures they elicit another reflexive expulsion: 'bless you' or words to that effect.

'Bless me' would be more medically accurate, as sneezes are a major transmission route of pathogens from the sneezer to anyone who happens to be in harm's way or touches surfaces that have been sneezed on and then – as we have learned is almost unavoidable – touches their eyes, nose or mouth. In this time of pandemic, sneezes are a major health hazard. If you must sneeze, do so into your elbow or a tissue.

In 2016, Lydia Bourouiba, a professor of fluid dynamics at the Massachusetts Institute of Technology, made a high-speed video of somebody sneezing.[23] This 1,000-frames-per-second movie revealed 'a turbulent cloud . . . of hot and moist exhaled air, mucosalivary filaments and drops'. The ejection phase lasted about 150 milliseconds and though the cloud had largely settled within half a second, some of the sneeze drifted around for several minutes and travelled 8 metres away from the sneezer. Please, please sneeze into your elbow.

The sneeze-disease link has been recognised for centuries. 'Bless you' is often said to have originated during the first waves of the Black Death in Europe in the fourteenth century, or perhaps during an even earlier outbreak of the bubonic plague. In the Roman plague of 590, Pope Gregory I is said to have ordered the recital of the short prayer *'deus te adjuvet'* (God help you) after every sneeze. Both explanations are unlikely, however, as sneezing is not a symptom of the bubonic plague, nor even of the pneumonic plague which occurs when the bacterium *Yersinia pestis* infects the airways. It probably dates even further back. Ancient Greeks viewed sneezing as a sign of good health and responded, 'May Zeus bless you.'

The nursery rhyme 'Ring a Ring o' Roses', with its sinister denouement 'atishoo, atishoo, we all fall down', is also widely believed to date back to the plague. However, folklorists point out that the rhyme itself did not appear until the late eighteenth century, the plague explanation was unknown until the mid-twentieth century and, again, sneezing is not a symptom of the plague.

What about the sex sneeze? I hear you cry. We will get on to that, but first let's deal with other non-tickly causes of sneezing. One is cold air, which can irritate the nasal mucosa and is probably why we call a viral infection of the upper respiratory tract a 'cold' – it mimics the symptoms of going out in wintry weather. There's also the photic sneeze, which occurs in response to sudden exposure to bright light. This afflicts about 20 per cent of people and is a genetic condition passed on by a dominant gene on chromosome 2, hence its other rather torturous alternative name, autosomal dominant compulsive helio-ophthalmic outbursts, or ACHOOS for short.

Exactly why it happens is a mystery, though the most plausible explanation is messy wiring in the brainstem. Bright light triggers contraction of the pupils, which is also a reflex action coordinated in the brainstem. Perhaps in some people unusual neural crosstalk accidentally triggers a sneeze reflex too. This may also explain another odd sneezing phenomenon called snatiation, or sneezing in response to a full stomach, and sneezing with a full bladder.

Any others? Remind me . . . Oh, yes, the sex sneeze. This first came to medical attention about a decade ago when a patient being treated in Slough by an ear, nose and throat surgeon called Mahmood Bhutta revealed that he went into uncontrollable fits of sneezing when he thought about sex.[24] Bhutta searched the medical literature and found some nineteenth-century case reports of sneezing triggered by sexual arousal, and one from the 1970s of a man who sneezed like mad after he had an orgasm. Bhutta's subsequent inquiries unearthed several hundred people who either sneezed during the inklings of arousal or after orgasm. About three-quarters were men.

Again, the most likely explanation is confused neural signals in the brainstem, which as well as controlling sneezing also trigger sexual arousal and orgasms. It is often said that sneezes are a sixth of an orgasm. For some lucky people, this turns out to be something not to be sneezed at.

4

Bad Guts

One of my favourite descriptions of the human body was coined by the American humourist Christopher Morley: 'an ingenious assembly of portable plumbing'. Indeed we are: from blood and lymph vessels to our airways, intestines and urinary tracts, a large proportion of us is dedicated to moving fluids from A to B.

In the biggest plumbing system of all, A is the mouth and B is the anus. Like most animals, we humans have what anatomists call a 'through gut'. That means it has a beginning, a middle and an end. Food and drink go into the mouth; faeces come out the other end. This is a far superior arrangement than is seen in some of our more primitive relatives. Jellyfish, anemones and corals have just a single orifice which handles both sides of the business. Polite society dinner party guests they ain't.

Between these two extremities lie an impressive 8 metres or so of tubes and chambers that are dedicated to extracting energy and other vital resources from food, and then packaging up and expelling the waste. But being so lengthy and complex, and coming into daily contact with material from the outside world, our guts are one of the most grumbled-about plumbing systems known to man.

There is an old saying in wellness circles that the road to health is paved with good intestines. For many of us a lot of the time, that is a pipe dream. But it pays to know the many disgusting and unpleasant ways your guts can go bad, if only to know how to avoid the worst. And remember that it could always be even worse: at least you have two orifices.

Hang on to your lunch, we are going in . . .

Halitosis

A certain member of my household has really bad breath, and I think I know why. He eats smelly food and never cleans his teeth. On a bad day his breath can make a grown man gag. But we tolerate it because he is furry, purry and adorable. I must take him to the vet to get his teeth sorted out.

Halitosis in a cat is acceptable. In a human it is a social death sentence. But as many as a third of people have chronic or recurring cases.[25]

The causes of bad breath are usually obvious: pungent food, poor oral hygiene and smoking. Others are less so. Some weight-loss diets can make breath smell awful, as can some underlying medical conditions.

The word 'halitosis' was coined by an American doctor called Joseph Howe in his vividly titled 1874 book, *The Breath, and the Diseases Which Give It a Fetid Odor, With Directions for Treatment*. He smashed together the Latin word for breath (*haltus*) with the Greek for disease (*nosus*) to create a total bastard that has been haunting humanity ever since. It entered widespread circulation in the 1920s when an obscure medical disinfectant company called Listerine – named in tribute to the British doctor Joseph Lister, who invented anti-septic surgery in the nineteenth century – repurposed one of its products as a remedy for 'chronic halitosis' and saw its annual sales rise from about $100,000 to $8 million. As one wag later said, Listerine did not so much invent mouthwash as it invented bad breath. (If Lister was unhappy about being rebranded as a mouthwash he was in no position to object, having obligingly died in 1912).

Today the market for mouthwashes, breath-freshening

toothpastes, sprays and breath mints is in the billions of dollars. The fear of halitosis has become a medical condition in its own right, called halitophobia. About a quarter of people who seek medical help do not have halitosis at all but have convinced themselves that they do. People with this delusional halitosis often become obsessed with teeth cleaning and oral hygiene in general and go to great lengths to prevent other people from smelling their inoffensive breath.

But if people routinely shrink away from you or turn their faces away from yours when you speak, halitosis is the probable cause. If you suspect you have halitosis, the easiest way to confirm it is to ask somebody who won't think ill of you to smell your breath. Self-diagnosis by breathing into a hand and sniffing it rarely works because people become habituated to their own stinky breath. Another popular method of self-diagnosis is to lick a wrist, let it dry, then smell the concentrated residue. But this tends to overcompensate and leads people to think their breath is awful when it isn't. A better method is to gently scrape the back of the tongue with a plastic spoon and sniff the residue.

The number one source of actual halitosis is an unclean tongue. Bacteria like its warm, moist, corrugated and nutrient-rich surface, and happily take up residence, especially at the back of the tongue where scraping them off is hindered by the gag reflex. A white tongue is often a sign of rampant bacterial growth. The bacteria break down food residues, saliva and dead cells and release malodorous volatile substances. These include the sulphurous compounds hydrogen sulphide, dimethyl sulphide and methanethiol, which give farts their eggy and cabbagey notes (see page 202). Bad breath is basically a mouth fart. But it is actually worse. Oral bacteria also produce stinky fatty acids such as butyric acid, which smells like rancid butter and vomit, valeric acid, which smells of over-ripe fruit, and vinegary propionic acid. Some leak out skatole, one of the signature odour components of faeces. Finally, there are the diamines cadaverine and putrescine, whose names tell you everything you need to know about how they smell.

All told, then, bad breath has all the charms of farts, sick, shit and dead bodies. No wonder we go to such great lengths to avoid halitosis and people with it.

The mouth also has numerous nooks and crannies such as the gingival crevices and periodontal pockets – the spaces between teeth and gums to you and me – which bacteria readily colonise. Unfilled dental cavities and the gaps between wonky teeth can fill with a bacterial buffet of compacted food.

The solutions to these problems are the standard tools of oral hygiene: toothbrushes, dental floss, tongue scrapers, mouthwashes and regular visits to the dentist.

Poor oral cleanliness can also cause a horrible taste in the mouth, though there are many other reasons why this happens. Colds, sinusitis, middle-ear infections, certain medications and acid reflux can also make your mouth taste disgusting, often strangely metallic. The human tongue can distinguish metallic tastes – think of blood – but this is usually swamped by other flavours. When the nasal cavity, which plays a huge role in flavour perception, is blocked or otherwise compromised, the metallic flavour can cut through.

Not all sources of oral halitosis will yield to standard oral cleanliness. Dental plaque – a layer of bacteria and fungi growing tenaciously on the teeth like barnacles on a rock – can be a source of fetid odours. Plaque also causes mild or severe inflammation of the gums, called gingivitis and periodontitis. Mouth ulcers smell bad. The worst-case scenario is called Vincent's infection, a.k.a. acute necrotising ulcerative gingivitis, which causes the gum tissue to ulcerate and die. It was common in the trenches of the First World War due to sporadic oral hygiene and general poor health; soldiers called it trench mouth.

Bad breath can also sometimes be caused by upper respiratory tract infections, infected sinuses, chronic tonsillitis or acid reflux. Foreign objects such as small pieces of Lego or dried peas lodged in the nasal cavity are another possible source, especially in children. These all require the attention of a doctor or dentist.

Not all halitosis originates in the mouth or nose. Consumption of spicy or strong-smelling foods such as garlic, onions, radishes, cabbage and cauliflower can lead to the metabolic production of rank substances that diffuse into the bloodstream and thence drift out of various orifices. That is why garlicky breath cannot be brushed or washed away. Some diets, especially low-carb ones, can also lead to the production of smelly metabolites that diffuse into the breath. The keto diet, which controversially shifts metabolism into starvation mode, is notorious for this. Its adherents may be svelte but also smelly.

Coffee and alcohol can dry the mouth and inhibit the normal salivary cleansing and so encourage bad breath; alcohol-containing mouthwashes can ironically do the same. Some women find that their breath sours when they are menstruating, again possibly because of dryness of the mouth. Good hydration is not just generally a good idea, but also a defence against halitosis.

All sorts of non-trivial diseases can cause bad breath, including diabetes, kidney and liver disease and cancer. Intractable and worsening bad breath warrants a check-up. Dogs can be trained to diagnose some forms of cancer from breath. Cats, not so much.

Bad breath in cats and dogs has the same causes as in humans. Some animals have even worse breath than my cat. A close encounter with a whale can envelop you in a cloud that smells of rancid fishy farts. In 1996, a safari guide called Paul Templer survived an attack by a hippo on the Zambezi River in Zimbabwe. The hippo half-swallowed him head-first; he later told reporters that its breath was absolutely rank, like rotten eggs.

Ironically, however, the animal that gives its name to bad breath does not actually have it, despite persistent rumours to the contrary. The Komodo dragon is often said to have a stenchy mouth teeming with bacteria that act like a venom, infecting the wounds of its victims and killing them by septic shock. This is a myth. Its venom is actual venom, and it mostly eats carrion (and hence probably has an extremely acidy stomach, see page 188).

Pretty much everyone has some level of dragon breath in the morning because the normal production of saliva, which helps to keep the mouth clean by flushing away food debris and dead cells, has been suspended during sleep. But morning bad breath usually goes away once salivary flow resumes and a cup of coffee or tea has been consumed and is not medically classed as halitosis. Breathe easy.

Hiccups

As a child growing up in the 1970s, I distinctly remember watching an episode of the after-school TV show *Blue Peter* which featured a girl who had had hiccups for months. She started one day and never stopped. Every time I got the hiccups after that, I worried that I too would be hiccupping for the rest of my life. It hasn't happened, yet.

The poor girl – I cannot find any reference to her on the internet, though my wife remembers the same episode – clearly had what doctors call 'intractable singultus'. If I remember rightly, she saw the funny side, but non-stop hiccups are no laughing matter. Fortunately, most bouts are short, often just a single 'hic'.

Hiccups are involuntary spasms of the diaphragm, resulting in a sharp intake of breath and the abrupt closure of the vocal cords and epiglottis, which produces the characteristic 'hic' sound. Many languages play on this and have onomatopoeic words for hiccups: the Dutch simply call them *hiks*, the French *hoquet* and the Spanish *hipo*. In Italian, however, they are *singhiozzo*, derived from the Latin word *singultus* which doctors still use as a formal name for this most informal of afflictions. Singultus is Latin for sobbing, and also death rattle. Hiccups are not worth crying about, nor fatal.

In Old English, they were delightfully called *ælfsogoða*, which means 'elf indigestion'. Along with many other afflictions, hiccups were thought to be caused by invisible arrows fired by elves. Some other folk traditions held that hiccups affect people when others are gossiping about them behind their back.

A handful of obscure languages feature voluntary hiccup-like noises called epiglottal consonants, which are produced by the sudden closure of the epiglottis. They include Dargwa, spoken in Dagestan, and Dahalo, an endangered language spoken by about 500 people in Kenya. I have not been able to find the Dargwa and Dahalo words for hiccups.

Invisible elf arrows and backbiting are no longer seen as plausible explanations. What is really going on is revealed by the fact that hiccups often strike during or shortly after a heavy or hasty meal, when a distended stomach irritates the diaphragm and causes it to spasm. The usual cause is eating or drinking too much or too quickly or swallowing air.

Dry bread is a classic hiccupy food because it ticks all three boxes: it is hard to chew so we tend to swallow big lumps along with a lot of air, and it makes us very thirsty. Food or drink that is either very cold or hot (in both senses) can also irritate the stomach and diaphragm, as can suddenly inhaling a lungful of very cold air. Laughing a lot can also make us swallow air and trigger a bout of hiccups. Pissed people hiccup because their stomachs are groaning with liquid and, often, gas.

Exactly why these largely harmless and often rather pleasurable activities – who doesn't like a piping-hot curry washed down with lashings of cold lager and a good laugh? – can trigger such an odd physical response is not known.

Several explanations have been put forward, largely inspired by the fact that babies hiccup a lot and hiccupping gets less common as we age. One very plausible idea is that it allows infants to expel swallowed air while suckling. The brief closure of the epiglottis shuts off the oesophagus and opens the windpipe, giving trapped air a window of opportunity to escape. The fact that other suckling mammals including cats, dogs, horses, squirrels and porcupines also hiccup lends weight to this idea.

There are other possibilities, however. Hiccupping actually starts before birth, as early as two months into a pregnancy, and expectant mothers can sometimes feel their baby hiccup. This has led to some other ideas about its function. Maybe it is breathing practice. Maybe it prevents the excessive inhalation of amniotic fluid. Or maybe it does not have a function, and is simply a relic of an ancient reflex which is reactivated during foetal development. According to this view, hiccupping evolved in a primitive amphibian ancestor as a rudimentary method of breathing. The classic combo of diaphragm contraction and epiglottis closure is still seen in some semi-aquatic animals that have gills, such as lungfish and tadpoles. The action draws air across the gill surface and hence allows oxygen to diffuse in and carbon dioxide out.

The evolution of fully functional lungs rendered this system obsolete, but as it is harmless and non-costly it was not selected against. In this view, hiccups are a bit like the appendix – a vestigial bit of biology that was once useful but now just lingers around and gives us occasional bother. The fact that premature babies whose lungs are not fully developed hiccup an awful lot is seen as further support for this idea.

Hiccups can occur singly, in bouts lasting from minutes to days, usually at a regular interval, or even for months and years. Hiccups that go on for more than forty-eight hours are called persistent; if they persist for more than two months they are intractable. Persistent and intractable hiccups can be debilitating; there are drugs that can help to stop the hiccups but they are sometimes a symptom of an underlying problem of the nervous system or gut. Anyone with persistent hiccups should go and see a doctor.

The world record for a bout of hiccups is held by Charles Osborne of Iowa, who started hiccupping at the age of twenty-nine and carried on for sixty-eight years. The cause turned out to be some minor damage to his brainstem sustained in a fall while hanging a hog for butchering. He did experience a brief respite in 1970 when his doctor tried out a new drug, but he did not like the side effects and decided that hiccupping was the lesser of two evils. His hiccups finally stopped in 1990, but he died soon afterwards. Osborne's hiccups stopped when he was asleep, but sleep hiccups are possible.

As for getting rid of regular hiccups, knock yourselves out. There are any number of folk remedies including giving someone a fright, putting cold keys down their back, drinking water from the wrong side of the glass, biting on a lemon, swigging vinegar, taking sips of ice-cold water, putting sugar under the tongue, exhaling hard with nose and mouth shut (the Valsalva manoeuvre, which is also used to equalise pressure in the ears), holding your breath, hugging your knees to your chest and breathing in and out of a paper bag. Osborne tried them all and more without success. There is scant scientific evidence that any of these do anything other than make you look a bit daft – hiccups are little more than an inconvenience and usually go away of their own accord, so not much research has been done, and almost anything can appear to get rid of hiccups if they happen to stop during the 'cure'. Unless the hiccups are getting in the way of something important you might as well just hic and bear it, and let them go away of their own accord. If you're still hiccupping sixty-nine years later, contact the *Guinness Book of Records*.

Food going down the wrong way

In 2010, a 75-year-old retired teacher called Ron Sveden was rushed to hospital in Boston, Massachusetts, with breathing difficulties. He had been diagnosed with emphysema a few months earlier and was getting steadily worse. He and his wife feared the worst, and when doctors did a chest X-ray they discovered that something was indeed growing in his lung. But it wasn't a tumour; it was a pea shoot about 1.25 centimetres long. Sveden had evidently inhaled a pea at some point and it had germinated in the warm and wet conditions of his lung tissues. The shoot was weeded out and a relieved, if slightly embarrassed, Sveden made a full recovery.

Inhaling food is surprisingly common, especially in children. Peas and peanuts are the usual culprits owing to their size and shape; some studies report that about 40 per cent of children aspirate a peanut at some point, many of them requiring hospital treatment to remove it. It is rarer in adults, but not unheard of. Around one in 100 adults end up in hospital having bits of food removed from their lungs, though most of them are not cultivating a plant down there.

As well as breathing in food, we sometimes make a mess of swallowing and end up sending it down the wrong way. Evolution has endowed us with two tubes in our thoraxes, the windpipe and the food pipe, but only one entrance, the nose and mouth. We have an elaborate system designed to keep food and drink from going into the lungs and air from going into the stomach but it is not foolproof. The latter mistake is pretty trivial; swallowed air turns into burps. But inhaling food can be big trouble. In the US, around sixty people – mostly children – die each year after a foreign body gets lodged in their lungs. But the vast majority of cases are resolved simply by coughing up the offending object.

Swallowing seems simple and effortless but is actually a complex process involving the coordinated action of more than fifty muscles. It is an automatic action, meaning that we don't have to think about it. But with such high levels of coordination required, a lot can go wrong.

Some people have chronic problems swallowing, often due to neurological damage from a stroke. Dysphagia can be a serious condition so we won't go there. But even people who can swallow normally occasionally get it wrong.

The main line of defence between food and the lungs is the epiglottis, a flap of cartilage in the throat which closes off the airways when you swallow. The uvula, which is the fleshy wattle hanging down at the back of your mouth and which is often mistaken for the epiglottis, also helps. (One of my favourite Far Side cartoons shows a perplexed medical student at the end of his final exam; the paper reads: 'Bonus question (50 points): what's the name of that thing that hangs down the back of our throats?')

But we still need to breathe when we're eating and drinking and occasionally our timing is off and food goes down the wrong way. Eating too quickly and talking with your mouth full can also glitch the system. Cue coughing, spluttering and gagging.

Pretty much anything in our mouths and throats can end up in the lungs, including food, drink, chewing gum, pills, saliva and stomach contents that have refluxed up the oesophagus (see page 187). That's right: you can be a little bit sick into your lungs.

The coughing reflex is almost always equal to the challenge but occasionally a solid object gets lodged in the airways and requires medical attention before it progresses to a severe cough or even pneumonia. Doctors will confirm its presence with a flexible camera called a bronchoscope, not unlike the ones plumbers use to peer into blocked drains.

They will attempt to remove it with long, flexible forceps but may have to resort to surgery. Talk about using a sledgehammer to crack a peanut.

Stomach ache, indigestion and heartburn

Food might be a glorious thing, but as the song from the West End musical *Oliver!* warns, overdoing it can have consequences. If you pig out on hot sausage and mustard, cold jelly and custard, pease pudding and saveloys, what comes next? Indigestion!

Indigestion is a set of mild and overlapping symptoms that commonly strike after eating too much and usually go away once the gut has dealt with our indulgences. They include stomach aches, heartburn, bloating, belching, nausea and sometimes that horrible experience of being a little bit sick in your mouth. Or a lot sick in the toilet.

The word simply means 'not digesting', but that is far too vulgar for doctors. They call it dyspepsia, which is a fancy Greek way of saying the same thing. But credit where it is due. 'Pepsia' broadly means digestion but has come to refer more narrowly to the stomach – as in peptic ulcers and the digestive enzyme pepsin. And indigestion is definitely a disorder of the stomach, usually caused by overworking it. All of the symptoms can be explained as a consequence of cramming in too much food, eating too quickly or guzzling grease.

Consider heartburn, which is a searing pain in the chest, often on the left side. It has nothing to do with the heart but is such a convincing mimic of a heart attack that about half of emergency room visits for a suspected cardiac arrest turn out to be heartburn. But doctors don't mind; better safe than sorry.

Heartburn may have nothing to do with the heart but it has everything to do with the burn. It is caused by stomach acid sloshing up through the cardiac sphincter – the circular muscle guarding the entrance of the stomach – and attacking the lining of the lower part of the oesophagus. Stomach acid is very, very acidic. If you extracted some and trickled it onto stainless steel, it would eat into it. The reason the stomach itself is not under constant acid attack is because it is (usually) lined with a thick layer of protective mucus. But the oesophagus isn't so blessed, and when it encounters acid strong enough to dissolve steel, it does not hold up well.

Why, you may wonder, is the stomach so devastatingly acidic? There are three reasons. Digestion is a long and laborious process which requires the conversion of big and complex biomolecules such as proteins, fats and carbohydrates into simpler ones that can be absorbed into the bloodstream. That is why the gut is so long and complex, with four separate compartments each carrying out a different part of the process. The stomach is compartment number two, following the mouth (which mechanically breaks down food through mastication and begins the process of enzymatic digestion of starch) and it has one main role: to get to work on proteins.

The ultimate goal of the digestion of proteins is to break them down into their constituent parts, called amino acids. That happens best under acidic conditions, which help to unravel tightly tangled protein molecules and expose them to attack by the stomach's protein-digesting enzyme pepsin. This has evolved to work best in strong acid. Acid also helps to kill off potentially dangerous food-poisoning microbes. And so our stomachs produce large quantities of hydrochloric acid, about 2 litres a day. As anyone who has studied chemistry knows, hydrochloric acid is a powerful acid.

Because the acid is a barrier against pathogens, animals that make a living by eating potentially contaminated food usually have the most acidic stomachs. A few years ago, a team of microbiologists reviewed the average stomach pH – a measure of acidity – of forty-three species of mammal (including humans) and twenty-five birds.[26] They found that the acidiest of all was the common buzzard, a frequent scavenger of carcasses, with a pH of 1.1 (the lower the pH, the stronger the acid). Vultures, carrion crows and albatrosses also have very acidy stomachs. Mammals tend to have less acidic stomachs, with some herbivores including llamas and sloths even straying into alkaline territory of pH 7-plus (pH is a logarithmic scale, so pH 2 is ten times as acidic as pH 3). But there were three outliers: ferrets, Australian possums and a great ape with the scientific name *Homo sapiens*. All have a stomach pH of around 1.5, more acidic than some carcass-scavenging birds. It is possible that some large mammalian scavengers such as hyenas, grizzly bears and wolverines have even lower pHs, but nobody has ever asked them, perhaps for obvious reasons.

For ferrets and possums that makes evolutionary sense, as both are frequent scavengers of rotten meat. But us? Surely we cannot . . . sorry, maybe we can. The researchers concluded: 'One explanation for such acidity may be that carrion feeding was more important in human evolution than currently considered to be the case.' Yep, we evolved to eat rotten meat.

That isn't a common diet any more, but one legacy of our scavenger past lives on in the guise of heartburn, also called acid reflux. When the stomach is very full, it makes more acid to deal with the huge influx of protein. The cardiac sphincter is also more likely to be under strain and hence leaky, allowing that strong, burny acid to bubble up into the oesophagus.

We do other things after a heavy meal that can make matters worse. Caffeinated drinks seem to loosen the sphincter, so after-dinner coffees make matters worse. But there is no link to alcohol. Which is a great excuse to pass on the coffee and go straight to a digestif such as brandy or port.

But go easy on that too. Leakage can also be gravity-assisted by lying down, or wind-assisted as the digestion process generates gases that escape as burps, carrying acid and partially digested food with them.

Greasy food also promotes acid reflux because it delays stomach emptying. The stomach normally does its work within three to four hours and starts to squeeze its partially digested contents into compartment three, the small intestine. But if it is swimming in fat the process takes longer, as the protein is harder to get at. Delayed emptying is also an adaptation to prevent the small intestine from being swamped. Fat is digested there but it only has limited capacity so the stomach acts as a holding pen. As a result, we stay fuller for longer, creating yet more opportunity for belching, acid reflux and a little bit of regurgitation.

Some foods are common triggers, though there is a lot of individual variation. The usual suspects are citrus fruits, tomatoes, onions, garlic, chocolate and peppermint, all of which have a relaxing effect on the cardiac sphincter. But not everyone gets heartburn after eating these, and some people have other triggers. My wife can't drink cider, which she blames on it being acidic. That is true but at pH 3–4 it is at least 100 times less strong than stomach acid, so that cannot be it. Ditto citrus fruits and tomatoes.

Overuse of non-steroidal anti-inflammatory drugs – aspirin and ibuprofen are the most common – can also make us susceptible to indigestion, as one side effect is to suppress the production of protective stomach mucus.

NSAIDs can also lead to generalised inflammation of the stomach lining, called gastritis. Stomach bugs, smoking and too much boozing can also bring it about. A classic symptom of gastritis is that frustrating feeling of becoming strangely full after eating just a small amount of food. Gastritis is the main cause of stomach aches, but by no means the only one. Constipation and trapped wind can also make your belly ache. It usually goes away in time.

Some people are prone to acid reflux and may receive an official diagnosis of gastroesophageal reflux disease. But the underlying cause is the same: gluttony. It just takes a bit less of it to trigger an acid attack.

Sometimes the stomach lining is breached, leading to a gastric ulcer. Once believed to be caused by stress or an excessively rich or spicy diet, we now know that the leading cause is an infection by the bacterium *Helicobacter pylori*, which neutralises stomach acid to create a less hostile environment for itself. This was famously proved in one of science's most spectacular stories of brave self-experimentation. In the early 1980s, an Australian doctor called Barry Marshall became convinced that decades of medical orthodoxy was wrong, and that stomach ulcers were caused by an infectious bacterium. He and his collaborator Robin Warren submitted a research paper claiming as much to the Gastroenterological Society of Australia, but were belly-laughed out of court. So Marshall prepared a broth of *H. pylori*, drank it, and quickly went down with the classic symptoms of a gastric ulcer, including bad breath (see page 176), nausea, pain, vomiting and inflammation. A biopsy showed that his stomach lining was infested with *H. pylori*. After two weeks of misery, he swallowed antibiotics and the infection cleared up, along with his symptoms. In 2005, Marshall and Warren were awarded the Nobel Prize in Physiology or Medicine. The Gastroenterological Society of Australia presumably ate a large portion of humble pie. Stomach ulcers are now largely treatable with antibiotics.

Regular acid reflux is also easily treated. The first line of attack is antacids, the simplest of which contain alkaline compounds that react with the hydrochloric acid in the same way that bicarbonate of soda reacts with vinegar. One of the products of this neutralisation reaction is carbon dioxide, so prepare to belch, which might just bring the problem straight back. For more troublesome cases there are more sophisticated antacids such as ranitidine, which dial down the production of stomach acid.

The other symptoms of dyspepsia are also caused by overeating, and the best way to avoid them is to go easy at the table. But food is so glorious that this is often easier said than done.

Nausea and vomiting

the other symptoms of dyspepsia are also caused by overeating, and the best way to avoid them is to go easy at the big meal of the day and to go for a quieter and duller time

If you're feeling a little queasy after the last chapter, you might want to skip this one. I don't want to make you puke.

Nausea and vomiting are one of the more unpleasant facts of life. But they are probably preferable to death by poisoning, which is why we have to put up with them from time to time. Most people vomit once in a while, though some people do it frequently and others almost never. My wife is a puker; I'm not. We generally eat and drink the same things and are exposed to the same bugs, so I can only conclude that she has a delicate and weak stomach whereas mine is made of cast iron.

But even non-pukers are queasily familiar with the sensation of nausea, which can strike without warning then fade, or build to its natural, horrible conclusion.

The sensation itself is the reversal of the normal mouth-to-anus muscular contractions of the stomach and intestinal tract, in part to return the contents of the small intestine to the stomach in preparation for getting rid of them.

Nausea is almost impossible to ignore; during a bout our horizons narrow and the world becomes a dismal place defined by waves of sickness, drooling, clammy skin, belching, retching and, eventually, vomiting.

For this horrendous experience we can blame evolution. Like pain, the distress of nausea and vomiting is a powerful warning to avoid in future whatever caused it. Animals that found vomiting distressing would probably have a slight survival advantage over ones untroubled by it, which is all natural selection needs.

Scientific interest in the causes of vomiting surged in the

1950s amid fears of mass radiation sickness after a nuclear war. Some gruesome experiments on cats and dogs established that vomiting was initiated by a patch of brain tissue in an area called the medulla, which is part of the brainstem. Electrically stimulating it caused the animal to vomit. Injecting emetic drugs caused it to fire up by itself, with the same end result. It became known as the 'vomiting centre'.

It was logical to think that humans had one too, and in 1962, doctors at the University of Utah discovered it.[27] They were attempting to relieve the misery of five patients with intractable vomiting due to inoperable brain tumours. As a last resort, they zapped the equivalent areas of their brainstems with an electrode, killing the nerve cells. All five stopped being sick and could not be induced to vomit by the drug apomorphine, which under normal circumstances is a grimly reliable emetic.

The vomiting centre is in the most primitive part of the brain, which is thought to have evolved in the ancestor of all vertebrates about half a billion years ago. It is thus reasonable to assume that vomiting is an evolutionarily ancient defence mechanism, and indeed palaeontologists occasionally discover lumps of what seem to be fossilised vomit (technically called regurgitalite, though inevitably dubbed 'Jurassic barf'). The oldest, recently discovered in Arizona, is 200 million years old. The vomit contains the bones of a dinosaur-like reptile called *Revueltosaurus* and was probably spewed up by another dinosaur-like reptile, possibly a rauisuchid, the dominant predator at the time. However, determining exactly which animal puked is not possible. (As David St Hubbins of *Spinal Tap* says, you can't dust for vomit.) Nonetheless, the cover star of the journal that reported the discovery is an artist's impression of a barfing rauisuchid.[28]

Rats famously cannot vomit, almost certainly because they lack the neural circuitry and their muscles are too weak. Nor can several other species of rodent – mice, voles, beavers, guinea pigs, coypus and mountain beavers (which are not actual beavers but a relative of squirrels). We know this thanks to a heroic research programme which tried and failed to make these animals puke.[29] The researchers who did it speculate that an inability to vomit is a general trait of rodents, but decided that testing all 1,800 species was 'clearly neither practical nor ethical'. Exactly why rodents have lost the ability is not known, but it questions the assumption that vomiting is a vital survival adaptation. An inability to vomit clearly hasn't held back the rodents, which are by far the largest group of mammals.

In cats, dogs, humans and, presumably, dinosaurs, the vomiting centre receives signals from four sources. The most direct of these is the gastrointestinal tract itself. The lining of the gut has sensors for ingested toxins and irritants such as food-poisoning bacteria and viruses that cause inflammation of the stomach and small intestine, otherwise called gastroenteritis (or stomach flu, though influenza viruses do not cause it). When these sensors fire in sufficient numbers, the vomiting centre initiates its ghastly programme and, if the signals go on for long enough, will eventually activate the vomiting response.

One of the most feared triggers of this branch of the vomiting system is the norovirus, or winter vomiting bug. This little swine is the most common cause of gastroenteritis and can curse its victims with repeated bouts of vomiting and diarrhoea over several days. It is horribly infectious. Somebody who ingests a single virus – a submicroscopic bundle of protein and RNA – has a roughly 50 per cent chance of going down with a bout. Noro is more unpleasant than dangerous, though, and usually clears up by itself. Though whoever clears up after you is probably next in line . . .

Another common cause of winter vomiting are the rotaviruses, which, if anything, are worse than noro. Rotavirus gastroenteritis usually announces itself with a bout of vomiting followed by several days of profuse diarrhoea (see page 198). Its R_0 number – the average number of people that an infected person goes on to infect – is off the scale, roughly twenty-five on average but as high as 190 in some outbreaks.[30]

Gastroenteric viruses are often spread via particles of vomit and faeces floating in the air or on surfaces, but can also be ingested in food. However, food poisoning is more commonly caused by bacteria, the usual suspects being *Salmonella, Listeria, E. coli, Campylobacter* and *Shigella*. They lurk in the usual dodgy places – undercooked meat, raw eggs, unpasteurised milk and cheeses, shellfish and out-of-date food – but can also be picked up from dirty water and unwashed fruit and vegetables. The first line of defence against them is our taste buds. If food tastes off or bad, throw it away, or you may well be throwing it up later.

If the bacteria get past your tongue, they can colonise your stomach lining and irritate it to the point of earning an eviction notice. Contrary to common belief, they don't produce poisons, so food poisoning is not really poisoning. Symptoms can start soon after eating the contaminated food but sometimes take days or even weeks to develop, as the stomach is searingly acidic and hostile to bacteria. Identifying what made you sick is therefore tricky. None-theless, you may well develop an aversion to whatever food you ate last before starting to feel bad. This is an evolved mechanism to learn from your previous mistakes, but can pick the wrong target and is susceptible to hacking. Memory researcher Elizabeth Loftus once did an experiment where she implanted false childhood memories of getting sick after eating hard-boiled eggs. Many of her subjects went on to develop an egg aversion.

The primary vomiting response can also be triggered by an overstretched stomach, perhaps from overeating or drink-ing too many pints (or both). Feasting Romans supposedly had a special room called a vomitorium where they could retire to throw up and make room for more. It's a funny and believable yarn but like many such stories is totally untrue; a vomitorium is actually a roomy corridor in the bowels of an amphitheatre that allowed the crowd to leave en masse after a performance. It sounds vomit-related because it has the same etymological root, 'to pour out'.

The vomiting centre also receives inputs from another structure in the brainstem called the chemoreceptor trigger zone (CTZ). This sits at the interface of the brainstem and bloodstream on the lookout for toxins. Their presence is a reliable indicator that a dangerous substance has found its way into the bloodstream, possibly from the gut, and that ejecting the contents of the stomach and small intestine would be a wise precaution. One such substance is alcohol.

Input number three is the balance system, comprising the motion-tracking vestibular system in the inner ear, vision, and sensors in the muscles, skin and joints called proprioceptors, which keep track of body position. If it detects any mismatch between these inputs, the brain makes the assumption that poisons have got into the brain and vomiting may be necessary. Alcohol can cause this too. It is also what causes motion sickness. The visual system tells one story – you are not moving relative to the boat, car or plane you are in – but the other two tell a different one. Cue hours of unrelenting misery.

Input number four is the cerebral cortex, the higher part of the brain responsible for conscious awareness, planning and other executive functions. This can be a powerful initiator of nausea and vomiting – you can literally think yourself sick. It can also suppress vomiting. In a remarkable magazine piece published in 2014, the editor of *The Atlantic*, Scott Stossel, came out as an emetophobe, meaning he had a pathological fear of vomiting that was ruining his life and career.[31] He finally agreed to treatment with exposure therapy, which meant submitting to an induced bout of vomiting. His doctor gave him a powerful emetic drug called ipecac, which makes most people puke. But not Stossel. He experienced horrible nausea and retching but he consciously fought it (as he had been doing for years) and managed not to seal the deal.

Extreme pain and fear can make some people throw up, for reasons unclear. Disgust is also a trigger, for more obvious reasons. This emotion evolved as a disease-avoidance mechanism; the physical recoil and classic screwed-up facial expression are probably designed to minimise exposure to potentially harmful substances such as rotten food, blood, faeces, dead bodies and vomit. It also activates the gag reflex, which is designed to eject foreign objects from the gullet. That is why the sight and sound of somebody being sick, or the smell or sight of vomit, can make us retch and puke. Even just reading about it can be nauseating, apparently . . .

And, of course, there's the old fingers-down-the-throat routine. This also triggers the gag reflex.

As well as initiating the vomiting response, the vomiting centre also seems to be involved in orchestrating the complex and rather balletic muscular movements involved in retching and vomiting.

It may seem a no-brainer that the stomach itself delivers the coup de grâce, but it doesn't. The final heave is actually created by your respiratory muscles – diaphragm, the intercostals between the ribs, and abdominals. These execute a series of violent spasms that cause retching and, ultimately, vomiting.

Postural muscles also kick into action to put you in the puking position – hunched over, head thrust forward, preferably into the toilet bowl (hence the expression 'talking to God down the great white telephone', as in, oh God . . . *bleaugh*) – to maximise the efficiency of expulsion.

Burping is a much simpler action. Accumulated gas activates stretch receptors in the stomach wall that cause the oesophageal sphincter – a circular muscle at the entrance to the stomach that is usually kept closed to stop semi-digested food and stomach acid from refluxing (see page 188) – to open. Physics does the rest; released from entrapment, the gas rises upwards and escapes through the mouth, vibrating the vocal cords on its way out. The gas can sometimes carry a bit of that semi-digested food and stomach acid with it, which is what causes those minor sick-in-the-mouth moments. This is also what will happen if, for some reason, you attempt to burp while standing on your head. The gas is not actively expelled but just follows gravity.

Anyway, back to the main attraction. The vomiting contractions can be so forceful that the vomit is hurled clear. This is the dreaded projectile vomiting that can sometimes strike with almost no warning if you get an especially virulent bout of norovirus. This lack of nausea followed by fountains of puke appears to be an evolutionary adaptation of the virus itself in order to maximise its infectivity. In one classic study, an outbreak of severe gastroenteritis in a British city was traced back to a hotel restaurant where a couple of weeks earlier a woman had suddenly and unexpectedly vomited onto a polished wooden floor. Staff efficiently cleaned up and the fine dining resumed. But over the next few days, more than fifty of 125 other diners who were there at the time started being sick, and the closer they had been sitting to the woman who threw up, the more likely they were to succumb. Almost everyone in her party fell ill, as did 70 per cent of people at an adjacent table. Even at the most distant table, the infection rate was 25 per cent. None of the guests reported actually coming into contact with the vomit.[32] Draw your own conclusions.

After two or three honks, you're done and the nausea will probably pass. If you're lucky, whatever made you sick has been jettisoned and that is the end of it. But more often than not it isn't, whereupon the nausea builds again and another bout of vomiting beckons.

This can happen even when the stomach contents have been completely emptied – for example, if the chemoreceptor trigger zone is still detecting the toxin in your bloodstream. Further vomiting won't help at this point, but, hell, better safe than sorry! This is what leads to the unproductive bouts of retching and vomiting called the dry heaves. It is also why being sick does not relieve motion sickness.

Even if nausea does not reach its natural crescendo, the experience is still pretty horrible. Physical discomfort can be exacerbated by emotional distress. This is the source of the cold sweats that often accompany nausea. Cold sweating is especially common during a bout of motion sickness.

The only sure-fire way to avoid nausea and vomiting is to never eat or drink anything, never spend time with other people and never travel on any form of transport. In other words, you can't.

But there are ways to minimise the risk, such as washing hands thoroughly (though be aware that norovirus is destroyed by soap but not alcohol hand sanitiser), being careful how you prepare food and what and where you eat and drink, and avoiding sick people.

If you share a bathroom with somebody who has a sick bug, ask them nicely to close the toilet lid after they have thrown up in it. Numerous studies have found that flushing a toilet with the lid up creates an aerosol of bog water mixed with whatever was being flushed away.[33] These 'toilet plumes' linger in the bathroom air and can also land on surfaces, where viruses such as noro can persist for weeks. They have been linked to disease outbreaks on cruise ships, aeroplanes and in restaurants.

Nausea and vomiting can have multiple causes, some serious, so if you suffer chronically or have frequent bouts, seek medical attention.

When you do become nauseous, there are some proven remedies. Doctors have extremely powerful anti-emetics at their disposal but you won't get your hands on them unless you have a debilitating and serious vomiting condition such as chemotherapy-induced vomiting. Some folk remedies such as peppermint and ginger have good evidence for their effectiveness, and some people report being soothed by sucking an ice cube or sipping fizzy water.

Ultimately, however, we have to accept that we vomit for our own good and suppressing it is not necessarily a good idea. So let nature do its worst. Better out than in.

Flatulence and trapped wind

In Kurt Vonnegut's novel *Galapagos*, a group of tourists is shipwrecked on an island in Darwin's archipelago shortly before a deadly new disease sweeps around the world (sound familiar?), leaving them the last surviving humans on earth. Over the next million years their descendants evolve into furry creatures a bit like sea lions. Not much remains of their humanity, except for one thing: 'If a bunch of them are lying around on a beach, and one of them farts, everybody else laughs and laughs, just as people would have done a million years ago.'[34]

Farts are funny and their humorousness is, believe it or not, a matter of serious scholarly debate. According to James Spiegel, a philosophy professor at Taylor University in Indiana, farts are one of the few universally humorous phenomena – meaning that they are funny in all cultures all over the world, for all of recorded history.[35]

But sometimes farts stop being funny. Some people endure the indignity of 'excess flatus' (flatus being the medical terminology for fart gas), either in terms of volume, or odour, or both. Others can't fart enough and get trapped wind. But before we get into that, it is worth boning up on some basic flatology.

Whether you admit it or not, you are a farter. Flatulence isn't just universally funny; it is universally human. Due to processes beyond your control, gases unavoidably build up in our large intestines and there is only one way out – the anus. As R.E.M. might have put it, Everybody Farts.

Most of the flatus is generated by gut microbes digesting carbohydrates that our own digestive systems cannot handle

– mostly complex polysaccharides, a.k.a. dietary fibre. The gas mixture is mostly hydrogen and carbon dioxide, plus sometimes a bit of methane. Hydrogen and methane are flammable, which is why you can light your farts, though this is not advisable as it can lead to a distinctly non-minor ailment, the burned rectum.

A small proportion of intestinal gas is not generated internally but is plain old air – mostly nitrogen and oxygen – that you swallowed but did not burp out and which passed from your stomach into your bowels and will now leave by the back door.

None of these gases smell of anything, let alone of farts (methane is also odourless; its distinctive smell is added artificially so that gas leaks can be detected). But microbial fermentation can generate small amounts of sulphurous compounds from sulphur in your diet, especially hydrogen sulphide, dimethyl sulphide and methanethiol. They smell, respectively, of rotten eggs, cabbage, and rotten cabbage. They are the principal reason why farts smell bad. Methanethiol smells so rank that it is sometimes used as an odorant for natural gas; a bad smell is more likely to spur people into action.

For good measure, farting also ejects volatile compounds found in faeces, notably skatole. This is the main smell of poo and is why some farts literally smell like shit – especially the so-called 'pre-dump pump' when your rectum is full of faeces.

Farts can be expelled silently; if they happen to be smelly they are colloquially known as the 'SBD', or silent-but-deadly. Large-volume farts can cause the anus and buttocks to vibrate noisily, producing the classic raspberry sound. Most people can do this deliberately and some even make a living out of this as stage flatulists – defined as 'entertainers . . . whose routine consists solely or primarily of passing gas in a creative, musical or amusing manner.' You may recall a flatulist called Mr Methane farting 'The Blue Danube' on a British TV talent show. He did not progress to the next round.

Farting, then, is both funny and revolting, but perfectly normal. According to the NHS, the average person lets rip five to fifteen times a day. And even if you suppress your farts, the gases will mostly just leak out anyway, a bit like a slow puncture.

But holding farts in is not a good idea. It increases the internal pressure of the rectum, which has been proposed as a leading cause of a painful and sometimes fatal inflammatory bowel disease called diverticulitis. This is most common in western, urban populations where fart retention may be more widespread due to social conventions about not pumping in public. And if that does not persuade you to let go, a held-in fart is partially reabsorbed into your bloodstream and exhaled. Fart breath.

We know what constitutes normal farting thanks to a landmark experiment in the field of flatology, performed in 1991 by a team of gastrointestinal doctors at the Royal Hallamshire Hospital in Sheffield. Their resulting research paper, 'Investigation of normal flatus production in healthy volunteers', was the first to establish a baseline of normal farting.[36] Ten volunteers – five men and five women – had a rubber tube inserted into their anus and kept there for twenty-four hours so their farts could be collected, measured and analysed, even as they slept. These hardy souls ate their normal diet, plus a 200-gram portion of baked beans to guarantee the researchers had some material to work with. They were allowed to remove the tube to defecate but had to re-insert it and seal it up with tape as soon as possible afterwards.

The volunteers produced a median of 705 millilitres of fart, with a range of 476 to 1,491 millilitres. There was no significant difference between men and women. Fart production peaked after meals but continued steadily across the twenty-four-hour period, including while the volunteers were asleep. Yep, you can sleep-fart.

The researchers then repeated the experiment on six of the volunteers (the paper did not explain why four did not come back) after feeding them a fibre-free liquid diet for the previous forty-eight hours, and found that their fart volumes fell to about 200 millilitres over the twenty-four-hour period, almost all of which was swallowed air. This proves, the researchers say, that the predominant source of fart gases is undigested food.

So much for normal farts. For some people it can all get too much. The NHS advises people to 'check if your farting is normal', which means an average of no more than fifteen farts a day and tolerable levels of smelliness. If either of these becomes excessive, or you have uncomfortable bloating (commonly known as trapped wind), it may be a sign of an underlying health problem. That includes the non-trivial conditions irritable bowel syndrome (IBS), pancreatitis and coeliac disease, which require medical attention.

But before going to see a doctor there are a few things you should try. Eat smaller meals, chew your food more slowly and exercise regularly to help your digestion. Work out which foods increase your fart volume or smelliness and avoid them. If you smoke, chew gum, drink a lot of fizzy drinks, eat hard sweets, habitually chew pen lids or have ill-fitting dentures, you may simply be swallowing too much air.

Some commonly prescribed medications can have flatulent side effects, including statins and anti-fungals. But talk to your doctor before dropping them. And beware of probiotics; although promoted as a route to good gut health, they more often cause flatulence than prevent it.[37]

If none of these work, your next port of call is a pharmacist. They can sell you pills made of activated charcoal, which soak up gases – anti-fart sweets, basically – or odour-absorbing pads or underpants. One leading fart-absorbing underwear brand (Shreddies: motto 'fart with confidence') claims that its activated-carbon back panel 'can filter odours 200 times the strength of the average flatus emission'.

For most people most of the time, farting is perfectly natural, normal and, let's face it, pleasurable. Not only is it funny, but people actually do like the smell of their own farts. In blind smell tests, many people find other people's farts repulsive but quite like their own. This is probably because farts are as individual as fingerprints and we find our own smells comforting and familiar. So stop holding it in and let rip.

Constipation and diarrhoea

One of my favourite-ever questions on my favourite-ever quiz show *Only Connect* asked contestants to find a link between the following four clues: 'like a sausage'; 'soft blobs with clear edges'; 'fluffy pieces with ragged edges'; and 'entirely liquid'.

The answer, in case you didn't get it, is the Bristol Stool Scale.[38] Invented in 1997 as a diagnostic test for bowel problems, it is also widely used by doctors to loosen potentially stilted discussions with their patients about bowel movements. The scale actually runs to seven categories; *Only Connect* started at Type 4 (the full entry is 'like a sausage or snake, smooth and soft'). For the record, Types 1 to 3 are 'separate hard lumps, like nuts (hard to pass); 'sausage-shaped but lumpy'; and 'like a sausage but with cracks on its surface'.

Types 1 and 2 (literally a Type 2 number two) indicate constipation. Type 5 is borderline diarrhoea; Types 6 and 7 are full-blown diarrhoea. The ideal stools are Types 3 and 4, which are soft yet strong (and sometimes very, very long) and hence easy to pass in one smooth bowel motion. I suspect that we've all been to every level at some point.

The word 'stool', incidentally, is thought to be derived from the non-scatological meaning of the same word, as in, a seat for one. The Old English word for 'throne' is *cyne-stōl*, which was truncated and vulgarised to mean an ordinary seat, then a seat with no arms or back, and eventually a toilet, the ultimate vulgar throne.

Both constipation and diarrhoea involve extended periods sat on the throne, either straining unproductively or exploding uncontrollably. It is hard to know which is worse, but let's start at the bottom, with Types 1 and 2. Stool consistency notwithstanding, constipation is difficult to define precisely as normal bowel activity varies a lot. Some of us routinely defecate more than once a day, others only three or four times a week. But if your stools are infrequent, hard, difficult to pass, and much bigger or smaller than usual, you have constipation.

The causes are quite simple and usually easy to resolve. The main culprit is a diet with too little fibre (that is why eggs are a classic bunger-upper; they contain almost none). Dehydration (see page 313) can also bung you up, as can lack of exercise. Eat more fibre, drink more water, lay off the eggs and booze and get off your constipated arse and you ought to be back in smooth sausage territory in a couple of days.

Bad toilet habits can also contribute. Postponing taking a dump when the urge takes you is a crap idea, as the longer faeces sits un-dumped in the rectum the more water is absorbed from it. Bad posture has also been blamed. Most westerners sit bolt upright on the throne with their feet flat on the floor, but a more natural position is the squat, which allows the rectum to straighten and relax fully and the stool to slide out easily. Sitting upright causes a kink in the rectum that makes it harder to completely evacuate.

One increasingly popular solution is the squatty potty, which is a footstool (the other kind) that raises your knees above your hips and unkinks the rectum. This has been shown to approximately halve the time it takes to perform a dump.

Some medications have constipation as a side effect, so it's worth checking the label of any you are on. But constipation can also be a symptom of more serious problems such as bowel cancer and diabetes, so if you are regularly bunged up, seek medical help.

If lifestyle changes don't work, laxatives probably will. There are two basic types – stool-softeners and muscle stimulants, neither of which really need any further explanation. They usually deliver the goods in a couple of days. One stool softener is a sugar alcohol called sorbitol, which draws water out of the bloodstream into the large intestine. It is found naturally in prunes and prune juice, hence the large market for both among the constipated masses.

Chronic constipation can lead to piles (see page 214) and faecal impaction, where solid stool builds up in the rectum. Strong laxatives or an enema usually sort this out but in extreme cases a doctor will have to excavate it manually using a lubricated, rubber-gloved finger. If you need a reason to eat more fibre or drink more water, this is surely it.

At the opposite end of the stool scale is diarrhoea, which, in case you have already expunged it from memory, is characterised by stools that are either fluffy pieces with ragged edges or entirely liquid. Diarrhoea often goes hand in hand with nausea and vomiting (see page 192) and has many of the same causes: food poisoning, gastroenteritis and food intolerances or allergies. Like vomiting, it often comes in repeated bouts and can last several days. You may also be treated to abdominal pain, bowel cramps and fever.

These symptoms are all geared towards the same goal – to expel the offending substances as quickly and efficiently as possible. The watery looseness, for example, is caused by a temporary shutdown of one of the large intestine's main functions, which is to absorb water from food and drink and reabsorb the water secreted into the small intestine. An average adult ingests about 2 litres of water a day, including the water in food; saliva, stomach acid, bile and other intestinal secretions add another seven. A healthy bowel will reabsorb the vast majority of this water, leaving about 100 to 200 millilitres to soften up those smooth sausages.

The presence of infectious bacteria and viruses inflames the lining of the gut and sends this system haywire. All that water stays put, and has only one exit route.

This is, in part, an adaptive mechanism to rapidly flush the contents of the bowels towards the exit door and facilitate thorough expulsion once they arrive. Nature's colonic irrigation, if you will. Abdominal cramping, meanwhile, is just an exaggerated bout of the normal muscular contractions that move bowel contents towards the rectum. That is also true of the explosive spasms that finish the job. Unlike vomiting, specialised muscular contractions are not necessary, just big ones.

It is worth checking the colour of your diarrhoea. Bright yellow can indicate a liver problem, black suggests a bleed in the small intestine and red a bleed lower down. All require attention. Green is usually okay, however, as it is usually just bile that did not get broken down.

Normal stools also vary in colour, from light brown through mid-brown to dark brown. Again, green is generally on the normal spectrum – eating lots of green food can colour your stools and is also a sign that you are eating lots of fibrous leafy vegetables. Very pale stools can indicate a lack of bile, which points to liver problems. Yellow is a worry for numerous reasons, especially if it is also very smelly. Red and black are possible indicators of bleeding, but if your poo appears blue there is probably something wrong with your eyes, not your bowels.

The Germans are very hot on interrogating their stools, and many German toilets feature a special viewing platform inside the bowl where the stool can be thoroughly examined before being flushed away.

If they need a visual aid, a variety of Bristol Stool Scale merchandise is available, from coffee mugs to mouse mats and T-shirts. Or, as the *Only Connect* team proved by getting the answer right after only two clues, they could learn it off by heart. Talk about knowing your shit.

Food intolerances

In my household we have a bit of a dilemma over hot and spicy foods. We all love them – the fridge has a dedicated section for chilli sauces and we usually have four or five different bottles on the go at any one time. But for one member of my household, who shall remain nameless to preserve her dignity, the ingestion of chilli inevitably leads to the violent expulsion of it from the rear end.

She has never been formally diagnosed, but I suspect she is among the approximately 10 per cent of people with irritable bowel syndrome, a loose and poorly understood cluster of gastrointestinal woes that include bloating, abdominal pain and diarrhoea. Attacks are often linked to the consumption of specific foods. Chilli is a common trigger; so are wheat and milk. But a whole shopping list of foodstuffs and beverages has been linked with dodgy guts, including fruit, pulses, cabbage, onions, peas, tomatoes, cucumber, processed meats, wine and beer.

People who have to hotfoot it to the loo after eating them are said to have a food intolerance. That term often produces intolerance among people hosting dinner parties, as well as some doctors who see it as a trendy, self-diagnosed ailment of the worried well. But anyone who doubts its existence is welcome to pop round to my house and listen at the bathroom door the morning after curry night.

One frequent culprit is the wheat protein gluten, which is also in oats, barley, rye and other cereals. Many people complain that eating bread and other gluten-laden foods causes bloating, gut rot, headaches, fuzzy-headedness, lethargy, joint pain, numbness in the limbs and rashes. This is commonly called gluten intolerance, though its official name is non-coeliac gluten sensitivity (NCGS). Anecdotally there is an epidemic of it – or at least of self-diagnosed cases – though its existence has not been established beyond doubt.

Some people truly are deeply intolerant of gluten due to a condition called coeliac disease. For them, the protein triggers an autoimmune response that attacks the lining of the gut. Coeliac disease affects around 1 per cent of people and can be the cause of serious health problems including malnutrition. In addition, a handful of people are allergic to wheat. If you have health problems that you suspect are triggered by eating cereals, the first thing to do is to rule out coeliac disease and wheat allergy.

To be clear: food intolerances are not the same as food allergies. The latter can lead to serious, life-threatening anaphylactic shock and require lifelong vigilance. Nobody ever died of a food intolerance.

As for gluten intolerance, studies have shown that some people have chronic gut-related symptoms that clear up if they go gluten-free. That may seem like an open-and-shut case for the reality of NCGS, but it doesn't rule out the possibility of a placebo effect, or that something other than gluten is responsible.

That something is often a group of carbohydrates collectively called FODMAPs, which stands for 'fermentable oligosaccharides, disaccharides, monosaccharides and polyols'. If you haven't got a degree in organic chemistry that is probably word soup; suffice to say that FODMAPs are carbohydrates that the small intestine finds hard to absorb, and so hang about in the gut being digested by bacteria. This creates large quantities of fart gas (see page 201).

Wheat contains large amounts of some FODMAPs (and lots of foods contain wheat) but so does a staggeringly long list of other foods: alliums, asparagus, artichokes (both globe and Jerusalem), beetroot, brassicas, cereals, fennel, fruit of all kinds, honey, milk, mushrooms, peas, peppers and pulses. And beer.

The worst offenders are onions, garlic, rye and barley – and wheat. So people who claim to be wheat-intolerant may be right, but for the wrong reason. Their problem is not gluten but FODMAPs. Going gluten-free also reduces FODMAP intake by about 50 per cent.

Around 70 per cent of people with IBS find relief by reducing their intake of FODMAP-rich foods. Cutting them out is so effective for IBS that the diet is now recommended by the NHS in the UK. However, going FODMAP-free is really hard. They are in so many foods that quitting them entirely doesn't leave much for you to eat.

Total abstinence is not necessary. The quantity and type of FODMAPs that trigger symptoms vary a lot between individuals, so many FODMAP-sensitive people only have to give up a few foods. Working out which ones can still be difficult. A lot of people start by quitting onions, and find that does the trick. Another approach is to cut out all FODMAP-rich foods then gradually reintroduce them one by one to see which are tolerable, obviously while keeping fingers crossed that one of them is beer.

A low-FODMAP diet is not necessarily a healthy one, however, because it rules out many foods that are rich in nutrients and fibre.

Another food that lots of people cannot tolerate is milk sugar, or lactose. This is down to genetics: their gene for lactase, the enzyme that digests lactose, is switched off in late childhood. This is actually the default condition of humans, but many of us now have a mutation that keeps the gene switched on throughout life. This mutation arose around 7,500 years ago in central Europe and spread quickly through the population, probably because it conferred the distinct survival advantage of allowing adults to digest a nutritious and calorie-dense foodstuff. Most people of European descent carry the mutation, but 90 per cent of people elsewhere do not. Intolerant people cannot break lactose down into smaller and more absorbable sugars so it hangs around in the colon and becomes food for gut bacteria. They guzzle it greedily and excrete gas, resulting in painful bloating, cramps and diarrhoea.

Chilli intolerance has also been linked to innate biology, specifically a higher-than-normal level of a pain receptor which responds to capsaicin, the hot compound in peppers. These receptors are found in the skin and also in the lining of the mouth and gut; their activation is what creates the hot sensation when we eat chilli. Intriguingly, the aforementioned anonymous female member of my family also sneezes uncontrollably if I happen to be frying chillies.

Most of the capsaicin we eat is absorbed into the bloodstream but some passes right through, as anyone who has suffered from a burned anus while dumping the remains of a spicy meal can attest. This is not what Johnny Cash had in mind when he recorded 'Ring of Fire'. Unabsorbed capsaicin can also cause receptors in the wall of the large intestine to scream out, leading to pain, cramping and violent expulsion.

The unnamed woman in my house also has a bit of a bowel problem with cabbage. We make our own kimchee, and we like it hot. Do not – REPEAT, DO NOT – come round to my house the morning after Korean night.

Piles

I don't recall which idiot told my dad this joke, but I do recall it going down like a lead balloon. What do haemorrhoids and BMWs have in common? Sooner or later, every arsehole gets one. At the time, my dad drove a BMW. The car had had one previous owner: my grandad. I'm not sure whether either of them ever had piles, but chances are that at least one of them did. The lifetime prevalence of haemorrhoidal disease is about 50 per cent.

The joke is therefore not just unfunny, it is medically inaccurate. But 'sooner or later, about half of arseholes get one' does not improve the punchline.

'Lumps in and around your bottom (anus)' do not sound good, and indeed they are not. This is how the NHS describes haemorrhoids, a condition commonly known as piles, though it quickly applies some soothing ointment. 'They often get better on their own after a few days.'

Haemorrhoids are a common problem of a surprisingly complex organ, the anus. They occur when, for reasons unclear, blood vessels in the anal wall become swollen or distended. About two-thirds of people endure them at some point in their lives, at least in the west. They affect men and women equally, though women are slightly more prone as they are a common ailment of pregnancy. People between forty-five and sixty-five are more likely to get them, as are the rich.

The word 'haemorrhoid' actually refers to a perfectly normal and healthy part of the human anatomy. The main function of the anus is to maintain faecal continence, or, to put not too fine a point on it, to stop shit from falling out of your arse. That system includes circular sphincter muscles and also a set of three structures called anal cushions, which are clusters of connective tissue, smooth muscle and a lot of blood vessels. These vessels are called haemorrhoids, derived from the Latin term for 'flowing with blood'.

And boy, do they flow. 'Perhaps the most singular characteristic of the anal lining is its great vascularity,' noted anatomist Hamish Thomson when describing anal cushions in a 1979 journal article.[39] The reason for this is to allow the cushions to engorge with blood in order to keep the anus firmly closed. They are also sense organs able to distinguish between solid, liquid and gas, and hence allow us to make the right decision with respect to letting go. Next time you fart with confidence, you can thank your anal cushions.

Sometimes these vessels become inflamed or even pop out of the cushion. These swollen or prolapsed haemorrhoids are piles. They can remain inside the anus or dangle out of it, looking not unlike a bunch of grapes, hence the nickname 'dangleberries'. They can be itchy, swollen and painful and often bleed after defecating or wiping. But they usually go back to normal after a few days. (Whoever coined the term 'anal cushions' seems to have had a rather warped sense of humour, because when they become inflamed they are the exact opposite of a nice comfy thing to sit on. It is possible to buy doughnut-shaped cushions that allow people with piles to sit comfortably.)

Piles are categorised into four grades depending on severity. Grade 1 are just swollen blood vessels with no prolapse. Grade 2 are prolapsed temporarily when straining on the loo – what is politely known as 'bearing down' – but spontaneously de-prolapse afterwards. Grade 3 stay prolapsed but can be pushed back in with a finger. Grade 4 are irreversibly prolapsed and may need to be removed by a doctor. The simplest way to do this is with a rubber band ligature, which strangles the pile to death in about ten to fourteen days. It then simply falls off, leaving a small patch of scar tissue. For really bad piles, surgery may be the only way to get them to leave your troubled behind.

Lower-grade piles can usually be avoided through dietary changes such as eating more fibre and drinking more water. There are also creams and ointments that can alleviate the discomfort. These usually contain two active ingredients – phenylephrine, which causes blood vessels to constrict and hence shrinks piles, and hydrocortisone, which alleviates itching. The skin-tightening effect of the phenylephrine has led to a popular belief that pile creams can also get rid of facial wrinkles. Kim Kardashian says so. But there is no scientific evidence either way.

Piles are often the butt of jokes. The satirical British comic *Viz* – never one to let good taste get in the way of a good joke – has a long-running cartoon strip called Nobby's Piles dedicated to a character with dreadful dangleberries, who invariably gets into scrapes that do not end well for his rear end.

If you think you have piles, perhaps because of blood in your stools or pain in your arse, they are easily recognised. The NHS supplies some useful, though quite eye-watering, pictures to help you – or somebody who doesn't mind looking at your anus, and vice versa – to self-diagnose.

If you do get them, console yourself that your anal discomfort has helped to save many more lives than it has blighted, thanks to the careful observations of an Irish doctor working in East Africa.

Denis Parsons Burkitt first went to Africa during the Second World War, serving in the Royal Army Medical Corps in the British protectorates of Kenya and Somaliland. After the war he set up a clinic in Kampala, Uganda, also a British protectorate at the time. He became interested in the widely different health problems of the indigenous and expat communities. One of the most glaring was in the incidence of piles. Burkitt reported seeing haemorrhoids galore among the expat community but rarely among his Ugandan patients. His observation echoed that of another British doctor, Hubert Carey Trowell, who had practised for nearly thirty years in Kenya and Uganda. He reported treating only two cases of piles in Africans, one of them a prince who had adopted a western diet.

Burkitt left a now-independent Uganda in 1966 and moved to England to continue his main research project on the cause of a type of childhood cancer that was common in East Africa. But he also maintained a keen interest in piles.

Burkitt hooked up with Trowell and, under his influence, began to think deeply about the wider patterns of health and disease he had seen in Africa. He noted that his pile-prone expat patients ate a refined, low-fibre diet whereas his Ugandan ones ate lots of roughage. He became convinced that the principal cause of piles was a lack of dietary fibre, which led to constipation and straining. This could forcibly eject a blood vessel rather than the recalcitrant stool.

At the time, piles were usually blamed on genetics, cold weather, sitting for too long on cold walls, tight clothing, vigorous exercise and even violent sneezing. Burkitt systematically ruled these out. On the genetic front, for example, he looked at data from the US that showed that piles were just as common in African Americans as European Americans.

Burkitt developed his pile hypothesis into a much broader and, at the time, radical claim about dietary fibre. He proposed that all sorts of western maladies including bowel cancer, heart disease, obesity, diabetes and appendicitis were caused or aggravated by a low-fibre diet.

Burkitt went on to write a best-selling book called *Don't Forget Fibre in Your Diet*. He was immortalised in a 1985 biography called *The Fibre Man*, which I suppose is better than being called *The Piles Man*.

Although the fibre hypothesis has largely been confirmed, its role in causing piles remains unproven. However, there are some established risk factors. Constipation is one, as is heavy lifting. Sitting on cold walls is not one of them, but sitting on the toilet for too long is. For this reason, the NHS advises against reading on the toilet. So put the book down . . .

5

Under Attack

One of my favourite-ever minor ailments cannot be found in any medical textbook and is not taught at any medical school: the lurgi. This magnificent term was invented by Spike Milligan and Eric Sykes for a 1954 edition of their radio comedy *The Goon Show* called 'Lurgi Strikes Britain', in which the country is battling a highly infectious disease called The Dreaded Lurgi. Again, sound familiar?

Lurgi quickly entered the lexicon as a catch-all term for an infectious but rather nondescript disease. Something a bit like a cold or mild flu that is enough to keep us off work but not bad enough to require medical attention. In other words, the quintessential minor illness.

Lurgi is not real, but there are plenty of bugs that are. Humans are fine pieces of meat and lots of things want a slice of us, from viruses and bacteria to fungi, intestinal worms and bloodsuckers. We are also big and scary and so many diminutive organisms have evolved elaborate defences to make us think twice about taking a slice of them. And sometimes our own defences turn on ourselves. We're endlessly at war. But if you are reading this, up to now you've won every battle. Long may it continue.

The common cold

In 1946, just after the end of the Second World War, a small military hospital on the outskirts of Salisbury, England, kicked off a campaign against a new enemy. Or, more accurately, an old enemy that had been attacking humanity for centuries: the common cold. It's a war we are still fighting and there is no end in sight.

There are lots of common diseases – this book wouldn't exist without them – but only one has 'common' in its name. It is very apt. An average adult catches four colds a year, and children six. We never seem to become immune and even though the symptoms are mild and usually clear up by themselves, colds are a serious burden on the healthcare system and the economy.

Colds are called colds not for the reason you might think, but because the symptoms resemble what happens when you are exposed to cold: runny nose, sore throat and shivering. The name dates back to at least the sixteenth century. In Shakespeare's *King Henry IV Part II*, Falstaff asks his young and sickly conscript, Bullcalf, 'What disease hast thou?' Bullcalf responds: 'A whoreson cold, sir.'

Almost inevitably, given the association between cold weather and common colds, the disease came to be seen as being caused by exposure to the cold. This 'you'll catch your death' theory persisted until surprisingly recently. It is mostly bunkum. There is some evidence that, for some reason, being cold can make you more susceptible to catching a cold. But being cold is not in and of itself a cause.

Anyway, back to the war. The campaign HQ was Harvard Hospital in Salisbury, a former American Red Cross field hospital for US troops fighting in Europe. In 1946, after the war was won and the GIs had gone home, the Red Cross handed it over to the UK Ministry of Health, which repurposed it as the Common Cold Research Unit.

At the time, the most basic scientific knowledge of colds was still lacking. Even medics widely believed the folk story that colds were triggered by getting cold and/or wet – draughts and wet feet were considered particularly dangerous. There was a fringe hypothesis doing the rounds that colds were in fact an infectious disease, but even those who advocated it couldn't agree among themselves whether it was caused by a virus or bacterium.

The unit set about trying to prove it one way or another. The unit's first director was virologist Christopher Andrewes, who had famously discovered the flu virus in 1933. He noted in a 1949 article in *The Lancet* that there was already good evidence for the infection hypothesis.[40] Some of the most convincing came from reports of remote communities where getting cold and wet was an everyday hazard but common colds were not. Bands of Arctic explorers, for example, were generally cold-free. In Spitsbergen, a remote outpost of Norway in the Arctic Ocean, colds were common in summer but not in winter – the opposite of what you'd expect if being wet and cold was the cause. In fact, colds usually vanished within two weeks of the last ship departing the archipelago in October, and reappeared in May after the ships returned. On the cluster of south Atlantic islands called Tristan da Cunha, meanwhile, cold outbreaks tended to happen after the arrival of ships from Cape Town but not from Panama, which suggested that they were caused by an infectious agent that fizzled out within a few weeks: the journey from Panama was long enough (more than twelve days) for whatever it was to infect everybody on board and then die out.

The Salisbury unit's early experiments were dedicated to testing the hypothesis that colds were infectious. Groups of thirty volunteers arrived by train on a Wednesday and were assigned to comfortable Nissen huts in groups of two or three; aside from the staff, these would be the only humans they had contact with during their stay. They were allowed out for walks but had to stay 30 feet (more than 9 metres) away from other people, which makes the 2 metres recommended for Covid-19 seem excessively familiar. On the Saturday they were 'inoculated intranasally', which meant having somebody else's snot or sputum dribbled into their nose. They then stayed for at least another week so the medical team could observe them and their colds.

By 1949, the scientists had established that colds were almost certainly caused by a virus. In 1956, they isolated the first such virus and called it rhinovirus – 'rhino' is Ancient Greek for 'nose'.

Between 1946 and 1990, when the unit closed, almost 20,000 volunteers passed through its doors. Thanks to their sacrifices and those of other volunteers and research groups around the world, we now know that there are at least ten major groups of cold-causing viruses, with a total of more than 200 different subtypes. New ones are still being discovered – in 2001, doctors in the Netherlands isolated a previously unknown cold-causing virus, the human metapneumovirus (hMPV), from nasal swabs of children with runny noses. And even the well-known cold virus groups can spring surprises. In 2007, a new type of rhinovirus – the most common of the cold-causing viruses – was discovered. There are probably many more still hiding under, or more likely in, our noses.

This incredible variety is the main reason why there is still no cure or vaccine for the common cold and why we fall ill repeatedly rather than developing immunity: it is not one disease, but hundreds. But hope springs eternal. More than 100 clinical trials of new treatments are ongoing.

A cure would be a major boon to the world. Even though colds are generally no more than an inconvenience and are usually eliminated by the immune system in a matter of days, they can exacerbate dangerous pre-existing conditions such as asthma and chronic obstructive pulmonary disease (COPD) and are a huge economic burden. Each year in the US, approximately 25 million visits to the family doctor are for colds, and colds cause 20 million days of absence from work and 22 million days of absence from school. During the Second World War, the UK Ministry of Defence estimated that absenteeism in munitions factories due to the common cold was costing the war effort 1,000 bombers, 3,500 tanks and a million rifles a year.

The most beneficial cure would be against rhinoviruses, which cause 30 to 50 per cent of colds. But the second biggest cause of colds, with up to 30 per cent of cases, is a category called 'unknown', which tells you how much we still have to learn.

Third is the coronaviruses, which shot from obscurity to global fame in 2020 thanks to their newest member, SARS-CoV-2. This appears to have jumped from bats or maybe pangolins into humans in 2019 and it remains a serious threat, as do two other recently emerged coronavirus diseases, Middle East respiratory syndrome coronavirus (MERS-CoV) and severe acute respiratory syndrome coronavirus (SARS-CoV).

But most coronaviruses cause only mild upper respiratory tract infections. There are four main strains, called OC43, HKU1, 229E and NL63.

All of them appear to have done a SARS-CoV-2 and jumped into humans from other species, mostly in the past 800 years or so. And like their more recent counterparts they initially led to outbreaks of deadly disease. Genetic evidence, for example, suggests that OC43 jumped from cattle into humans in the nineteenth century and caused a deadly pandemic of a previously unknown respiratory disease in 1889. NL63, meanwhile, probably first infected people between the thirteenth and fifteenth century. But as often happens with new viruses, they evolved to be less deadly. This happens for two main reasons: viruses that kill their hosts too quickly are shooting themselves in the foot, and people who happen to be highly susceptible are permanently removed from the gene pool.

Some other non-coronavirus cold bugs also started life as deadly pathogens that became less virulent with time. Rhinovirus C, for example, emerged 8,000 years ago, around the time that people began to settle in villages, and was a major killer of children.

That may well be what eventually happens to SARS-CoV, MERS-CoV and SARS-CoV-2: they become just another cold virus that bugs us from time to time. But that will not happen for a long time.

The four common-cold-causing coronaviruses, incidentally, have another dastardly trick that helps to explain why we constantly get colds, never seem to become immune, and have failed to develop a vaccine. For some reason the human immune system does not appear to generate long-term immunity to them, which means that, unlike many other viruses (think measles and chickenpox), we can catch the same one again and again.

Up to 15 per cent of colds are actually mild influenza, so are technically not a cold at all. There's also a cast of minor characters that each cause 5 per cent or fewer cases: respiratory syncytial viruses, parainfluenzas, adenoviruses, enteroviruses, metapneumoviruses, bocaviruses and polyomaviruses. But don't worry too much about those; there isn't an end-of-chapter exam.

You catch a cold mainly by breathing in fine droplets of virus-laced bodily fluids that have been sneezed or coughed out by an infected and symptomatic person. Every day we inhale about 15,000 litres of air – enough to fill about 500 party balloons – some of which has recently been coughed or sneezed out by other people. That's correct: you constantly inhale other people's snot and spittle.

These snot and spit aerosols hang in the air for hours and can spread several metres from their source, especially indoors where there is no wind to disperse them. They also settle on surfaces and can linger there for days. If you touch a contaminated surface – technically called a 'fomite' – and then touch your nose or mouth, you can transfer the virus to where it wants to be, the inside of your respiratory tract. Infections are also passed on by a direct hit of large droplets from an unshielded cough or sneeze.

This is one reason why colds are more common in the winter – we spend more time indoors, huddled close to other people, breathing in their sneezes and coughs, being coughed and sneezed on directly and touching disgusting surfaces.

This is also why colds have evolved to make you sneeze and cough: airborne transmission is a very effective way of selecting a new victim and hence breeding the next generation of cold viruses. Think of your sneezes as viruses having sex (not too much of a leap of the imagination – sneezing has been likened to a mini-orgasm anyway).

The viruses don't know to make you sneeze and cough, of course. Natural selection has simply eliminated viruses that happen not to spread efficiently, which means those with an R_0 number of less than one. The R_0 number is the 'reproduction number', the average number of other people that somebody with an infectious disease infects. You may recall from the pandemic that an R_0 number of greater than one leads to exponential growth of cases, as each infected person infects more than one other. The R_0 number of common cold viruses is typically between two and three, which is quite low – the measles virus has an R_0 of fifteen or more – but high enough to keep the disease circulating constantly.

Once the virus has wheedled its way into its next victim's nose or mouth, it invades cells in the surface epithelium and commandeers them as virus factories, churning out yet more viruses that spread rapidly through the upper respiratory tract – the nasal cavity, pharynx, larynx and upper trachea (windpipe). Cold viruses don't usually infect the lower trachea and lungs, which is a major difference between colds and flu.

The symptoms of colds and flu are very similar, but flu is usually much worse. In the 2019–20 flu season in the US, for example, of the 38 million people who caught the virus, 405,000 required hospitalisation and 22,000 died.[41] Influenza is not a minor ailment, so we will say no more about it.

Around 25 per cent of cold virus infections pass off without causing illness. Those that progress do so rapidly, with symptoms usually appearing no more than twelve hours after infection. The first hint that you've got a cold coming on is a sore throat, which is caused by inflammation of the tissues on the inner surface of the pharynx (see page 160). This usually goes away quickly but by then you've also got the other all-too familiar symptoms: runny and stuffy nose, sneezing, cough, fever, headache and lassitude. Muscle aches also happen, though are less common than in flu (I said I wasn't going to mention that again, dammit).

Of these, most patients find stuffiness and nasal discharge the most bothersome. The symptoms worsen rapidly, peaking within three days of infection, and then dwindle away as the immune system does its stuff. The average duration of a cold is seven to ten days, but they can linger for three weeks.

You may curse the virus, but they don't actually do you much direct harm. Most of the symptoms of a cold are caused by the body's response to it. A runny nose, for example, is an attempt to flush the virus out. The dense and more purulent snot that bungs you up later is thickened and made yellowy-green by the bodies of white blood cells that have sacrificed themselves for you. Fever, meanwhile, is the immune system's way of creating a hostile environment for viral invaders, which function best at normal body temperature. Muscle aches are another side effect of the immune response, caused by inflammatory compounds such as interleukins.

The immune response to an infection also triggers what is called 'sickness behaviour': retiring to bed, sleeping a lot, avoiding food and losing interest in social interaction. These are thought to be evolved responses to speed recovery and prevent us from passing the pathogen on.

There is no cure for the common cold but the symptoms can be eased, a bit. In 2018, the *British Medical Journal* rounded up all the evidence in an article called 'What treatments are effective for common cold in adults and children?'[42] Its conclusion: not many.

The article looked at three common symptoms: runny nose, stuffiness and sneezing. It concluded that your best bet for relief of all three without side effects is a combination of an anti-inflammatory antihistamine, a painkiller and a decongestant. But the evidence base was deemed low quality, and children under twelve should not be given decongestants as they don't work and may be harmful.

The list of things that don't work is long and, if you are a pharmacist or health-food retailer, a huge business opportunity. They include Chinese herbal medicines, echinacea, eucalyptus oil, drinking lots of fluids, garlic, ginseng, honey, probiotics, vapour rubs, vitamin C and zinc. Antibiotics do not kill viruses and are positively harmful.

The old adage that we should 'feed a cold' is based on that obsolete belief that colds were caught by getting cold, and that a hot meal would warm us up and hence cure it. If anything, colds should be starved; research on mice suggests that infections caused by viruses get better faster when they are fasting. The other half of that adage is also wrong; starving a fever is possibly the worst thing you can do. If anything, we should starve a cold and feed a fever (for more on fevers, see page 236).

On the upside, there are things we can do to minimise our risk of getting a cold in the first place. Many became familiar during the Covid-19 pandemic. Keep your distance from other people, wash your hands frequently with soap and water, avoid touching surfaces, don't touch your nose and mouth, wear a face mask. Vitamin D supplements can help too, especially in the winter. The vitamin is a general immune-system booster but people tend to become mildly deficient in it towards the end of winter. That is because the main source is ultraviolet light hitting uncovered skin, which stimulates the conversion of a common dietary compound into vitamin D. However, at latitudes north of Madrid and San Francisco and south of Melbourne, Australia, the winter sun is not strong enough to trigger this reaction and the body's stores of vitamin D start to run low. Vitamin D supplements are a very good way of topping them up and are a wise defence against colds and other cold-season infections such as the flu.

Failing that, you could always consider overwintering in Spitsbergen. Just don't forget your vitamin D.

Bronchitis and wheeziness

An upper respiratory tract infection or URTI can sometimes penetrate deeper into the airways, developing into an LRTI. (There are also MRTIs but they are usually called by their other names, laryngitis and pharyngitis, see page 160. These can also creep down the windpipe and develop into LRTIs.) An LRTI is formally known as bronchitis because its main feature is inflammation of the bronchi, the larger airways inside the lung itself. These begin where the trachea bifurcates and continue down to the fifth or sixth bifurcation.

Bronchitis is commonly known as a chest infection or chest cold. And that, indeed, is what it usually is. The most common cause – at least of the acute version, which lasts no more than a couple of weeks – is one or other of the common cold viruses that has strayed beyond its usual domain in the upper respiratory tract, down into the lower one. Flu viruses also do this, though as we have seen the distinction between cold and flu viruses is not a clean one. About 10 per cent of cases are caused by bacteria. Acute bronchitis is very common, though nowhere near as common as the common cold. About one in twenty people suffer a bout each year.

The most obvious symptom of bronchitis is a deep, wet, hacking cough (see page 163), which is the body's attempt to eject the mucus that has built up in the airways due to the ongoing battle between the immune system and the invader. Wheezing and rasping are products of this too, the sound of air struggling to get past partial blockages of mucus. Which is why a good, productive cough can put a stop to them.

The immune system usually wins the battle, though in cases of bacterial bronchitis may need help from antibiotics.

As with colds versus flu, the boundary between upper and lower respiratory tract is also often the boundary between minor and major disease. Acute bronchitis, especially the bacterial one, can creep right through one or both lungs, at which point it becomes the life-threatening disease called pneumonia. In medical circles this has long been known as the 'old person's friend' because it is a swift and relatively painless way to die.

Chronic bronchitis, classed as bronchitis lasting for a minimum of three months for at least two years, is usually caused by smoking. Don't smoke.

Swollen glands

My wife is a frequent sufferer of swollen glands. If she is even a little bit ill with a sniffle or cough, small squishy lumps appear under the skin in her neck and armpits and inflict uncomfortable aches and pains. Sometimes they do this to her even if she is not noticeably ill. She considers these inflamed glands a sign that she is about to be struck down. It reminds me of the old saying about the hills and the rain: if the glands are not swollen, you're going to ail. If they are swollen, you're already ailing.

Except that her glands are *not* swollen, because they are not glands. By definition, a gland has to synthesise and secrete something, such as sweat, hormones, saliva or milk. The bean-like structures in our necks, armpits and groins that swell and become tender when we are ill are actually lymph nodes. They are an important and interesting feature of human anatomy. But they are not glands.

The lymphatic system is one of the human body's unsung heroes. Often regarded as little more than a drainage network, it is much more important than that. And yet until recently it was a neglected feature of anatomy, often taking a back seat to its more glamorous other halves, the circulatory and immune systems.

As blood travels around the body dropping off oxygen and nutrients and picking up waste products, some of the fluid portion – called plasma – inevitably leaks out into tissues where it becomes known as interstitial fluid. It is a precious resource that needs to be returned to the bloodstream, and this is primarily what the lymphatic system is for. It is basically a network of tubes that collect leaked fluid (which, once captured by the lymph system, is rebranded as lymph) and deliver it back to the jugular vein, where it rejoins general circulation.

It is more than mere plumbing, however. For one thing, it carries fats absorbed from the digestive system into the bloodstream (other nutrients go straight in). It also returns immune cells that have wriggled out of the blood vessels to attack invaders, or at least the ones that lived to tell the tale. It collects toxins and gubbins including the remains of those brave immune cells to be dumped into the bloodstream and filtered out by the kidneys. But by far its most vital function is immune surveillance.

All the way along the estimated hundreds of kilometres of lymph vessels are lymph nodes. There are around 450 such nodes in a human body, clustered around (though by no means confined to) the groin, armpits, neck and head. They are shaped like kidney beans up to 2.5 centimetres long. Their job is to act like immune checkpoints, scanning the lymph for danger as it flows back towards the bloodstream.

Many of the bacteria and viruses that invade the human body initially get into the tissues rather than the bloodstream itself, so the lymph system is an important entry point for pathogenic organisms. Viruses and bacteria that are busy attacking the respiratory tract, tonsils or other warm and wet internal surfaces can also get swept into the lymph system.

When pathogens arrive at a lymph node, they are in for a hostile reception. Each node has afferent vessels, which deliver lymph, and efferent vessels, which take it away again. While the fluid is in the node it is filtered through a mass of immune cells. If one of them encounters a virus or bacterium, it launches a swift and usually fatal (for the invader) attack.

Immune cells in the node can also proliferate in response to a major invasion – of the node itself or a nearby tissue – and this is what causes them to swell. Inflammatory responses also kick in, which add to the swelling, technically called lymphadenopathy. This is why upper respiratory tract infections are often accompanied by swollen nodes in the neck: they are pumping out immune cells to help fight the infection. Circulating immune cells can also come to an infected node's rescue, further packing it with white blood cells, both living and dead (a.k.a. pus).

Swollen lymph nodes are therefore a sign of an ongoing immune response to an infection, which is almost always a good sign. The most common triggers of swollen nodes are coughs and colds, ear and throat infections, tooth abscesses and infected wounds. They are also one of the main symptoms of infectious mononucleosis, often called mono, which is why that common viral infection was once widely known as glandular fever (see page 248). They usually return to normal in a week or two.

If they don't, and/or are unusually large, hard and painful, they may be a sign of something more serious. Some autoimmune diseases and HIV can cause the nodes to swell. Cancer cells can travel around the body in the lymph system; they sometimes lodge in the nodes and start proliferating. If swollen lymph nodes are troubling you, the advice is to consult a doctor. Just don't describe your symptoms as swollen glands.

Fever

As warm-blooded animals, we humans are experts at maintaining a roughly constant internal temperature. However hot or cold it is outside, our insides generally bump along at around 37°C, or 98.6 degrees Fahrenheit in old money. The exact number varies a bit from person to person, in different parts of the body, between men and women (women are, on average, slightly hotter, especially in the second half of the menstrual cycle) and through the day, but a core temperature of anything between 36.5°C and 37.5°C is considered normal.

But from time to time, our bodies whack up the thermostat. Once the internal mercury hits 38°C (100.4°F), we are said to be running a fever, or pyrexia. At 40°C we have entered a medically dangerous state called hyperpyrexia.

Fevers are usually triggered by infections such as flu, common colds and, of course, our new public enemy number one, Covid-19. As long as they stay under 40°C they are an indication that the body is fighting back successfully. High temperature is one of the immune system's key defences against pathogens, as it both interferes with the biological functioning of some viruses and bacteria and speeds up some of the immune system's critical chemical reactions. It appears to be an evolutionarily ancient response: cold-blooded animals such as lizards attempt to soak up more heat than normal when they have an infection.

The human body generates most of the excess heat internally. It achieves this by temporarily recalibrating the central thermostat in a brain area called the hypothalamus. This essentially tricks the body into thinking it is too cold, causing it to ramp up the furnaces like it does when we are outside on a cold day. This is the source of the chills and shivering that can paradoxically accompany a fever: body temperature may actually be way above normal but, according to the recalibrated thermostat, feels like it is below. This further ratchets up the fever in two ways: shivering muscles generate heat, and the subjective feeling of cold can promote heat-conserving behaviours such as crawling under the duvet with a hot water bottle. Like lizards, we seek out heat when under the weather. But this can cause an overshoot, and we suddenly feel like we're burning up. Hence the feverish cycle of chills and sweatiness. They can even occur simultaneously as we cycle from one to another, which partly explains the feverish paradox of the cold sweat. Cold sweating, defined as sweat production without an increase in body temperature, can also be induced by psychological stress, such as nausea (see page 199).

Mild fevers do not need to be treated, and doing so can actually inhibit the immune response and delay recovery. But only a bit, so if the fever is uncomfortable, anti-inflammatory drugs such as paracetamol and ibuprofen should help. Cool drinks can also lower core temperature, but soothing damp cloths on the forehead are too peripheral to have any real effect.

As for the old adage that you should starve a fever, it has no basis in medical science – research on mice suggests that bacterial infections (which are more likely to make us feverish) clear up quicker when well fed. If anything, it makes sense to eat more: the excess heat of a fever is created by throwing more fuel on the metabolic fire, which burns a lot of energy. A 1°C rise in body temperature requires a 10 per cent increase in metabolic rate. So scoff away. But don't worry if you can't face food. There's plenty of energy stored away in fat and muscle to keep the fires burning.

If a fever reaches 40°C, seek medical help. Hyperpyrexia can lead to organ failure and even death. The most accurate way to measure core temperature is to shove a thermometer up your bum. Mouths and armpits are a bit cooler. And be careful of putting a thermometer in your mouth anyway; you don't know where it has been.

Light-headedness

One common symptom of being under attack from viruses or bacteria is light-headedness – a vague feeling of floating, as if your head has turned into a balloon, combined with dizziness, vertigo, tunnel vision, disconnection from reality and, ultimately, passing out.

This rather weird sensation is usually caused by nothing worse than dehydration. Water loss is a hazard of sick bugs, for obvious reasons, but any infectious disease can push our water balance out of whack. Runny noses, coughs and sweating are direct drains on our fluid reserves, but loss of appetite can also cause stealth dehydration as about 25 per cent of water intake normally comes from food. Some foods are obviously very watery – watermelon, for example, is about 90 per cent water. But even some very dry foods are secretly quite wet. Bread is about 40 per cent water.

Dehydration makes us woozy because it causes blood volume to drop and hence blood pressure to fall. This hypotension (which is easily confused with hypertension, or high blood pressure, but is of course its exact opposite) reduces blood flow to the brain, which starves it of oxygen and stops it from working properly. We subjectively experience this as light-headedness.

Hypotension is also the reason why standing up too quickly can make us feel faint. The blood cannot keep up, and our brains experience a brief bout of what is called postural, or orthostatic, hypotension. Orthostasis is an unnecessarily complicated word meaning 'to stand up.'

Low blood sugar can also interfere with brain function – the brain is a metabolically very expensive organ even when it is doing nothing except lying ill in bed – and has a voracious appetite for both oxygen and glucose. A fired-up immune system is also a guzzler of energy, and in this wartime economy everything else, including the brain, has to go on meagre rations to support the troops.

If the dehydration and/or starvation of the brain all gets too much, it eventually shuts down and we lose consciousness. Fainting is a survival mechanism. It temporarily reduces the brain's demands for oxygen and glucose and, by making us slump to the floor, can help to improve blood flow to the head. Faints usually last no more than twenty seconds.

The medical term for fainting is syncope, which is rather pleasingly derived from a Greek expression meaning 'to cut off the sun'. The sun itself can cause us to faint. If we overheat, peripheral blood vessels dilate to help cool the vital organs. This can cause blood pressure to drop, and the walls to close in. Tunnel vision is a common experience during presyncope – the prelude to fainting. It is another subjective experience of the objective fact that the brain is shutting up shop for a while.

The combination of dehydration and low blood sugar is, of course, a great marketing opportunity. In 1927, William Hunter, a pharmacist from Newcastle upon Tyne, invented a drink called Glucozade, which was basically carbonated sugar water with a vaguely medicinal citrus flavour (it was also a bit of a swizz under the Trade Descriptions Act, as the sugars in it were not glucose but dextrose and maltose). In 1938, the drug company Beecham's bought the recipe, rebranded it 'Lucozade' and started selling it as a recovery drink for the sick. It was a huge success; Lucozade was sold in pharmacies and generations of British kids feigned illness in the hope of getting their sticky mitts on a bottle. In 1953, Beecham's built a Lucozade factory next to the M4 motorway in Brentford, West London, and adorned it with an illuminated kinetic billboard proclaiming 'Lucozade Aids Recovery'. It won a cult following and in 2016 the company – which had by then been swallowed up by the international pharma giant GlaxoSmithKline, which itself had offloaded the Lucozade brand in 2013 – was on the receiving end of an unanticipated public backlash when it took the sign down and demolished the factory. The iconic billboard is now on display at the nearby Gunnersbury Park Museum.

Dizziness can also be caused by ear infections, which can play havoc with the balance system and induce a feeling of vertigo (see page 139). This is also the reason why going on a waltzer or similar angular-momentum-based fairground ride induces dizziness: the fluid in the vestibular system that helps to detect our direction of motion continues to slosh around, making it seem as though your head is still spinning.

Another classic fainting cue is blood. This is a real thing – about 15 per cent of people feel faint or actually pass out at the sight of blood. For some people, merely thinking about blood can cause a wobble. Needles do the same to some people. Evolutionary psychologists, who seldom pass up an opportunity to explain away curious human behaviours as adaptations that would have been useful to our distant ancestors, have proposed that fainting at the sight of blood is a form of 'playing dead', which some other animals do to deter would-be predators or attackers.

If you do feel faint, the old advice is the best: sit down and put your head between your knees. This is also a useful position to be in if you do actually faint, as there is less far to fall. Fainting is a major cause of head injury and concussion. Talk about adding injury to insult.

Chickenpox and other childhood diseases

Back in my undergraduate days I lived in a rather chilly and dismal flat above a greengrocer's shop in south-west London. One Easter break I went back to my parents' to take advantage of their well-stocked fridge, mould-free bathroom and central heating. My flatmate (not the sex-sneeze one) decided to stay in London to revise for his exams. The bloody swot. He didn't get much work done.

After Easter I went back to London and discovered that the flat had been occupied by a monster. It was huddled in bed wearing only a soiled dressing gown, with matted hair and hideous lesions all over its face. On closer inspection it turned out to be my flatmate, struck down with a very nasty bout of chickenpox. This was pre-internet days and the only people who had mobile phones were yuppies in the city. Our flat had a landline but it was for incoming calls only. Our landlord, who ran the shop below, didn't trust us to pay the phone bill. Ironically, he was eventually the one who did a runner, for reasons we never discovered. I hope it was an unpaid phone bill.

My flatmate was absolutely riddled with the pox. He had spots all over his scalp and face, in his mouth, on his eyelids and in various places where the sun don't shine (I took his word for that). He had not had chickenpox as a child and, like many people who get it later in life, had it very bad. He said he had written me a letter warning me not to come back if I hadn't had the pox (I had, very mildly, and did not catch it myself) but by the time he finished it he was too unsightly to venture out to the post office.

Chickenpox is one of those rites-of-passage diseases that pretty much everyone gets sooner or later – preferably sooner, as it generally produces milder symptoms in young children.

When I were a lad, you were also expected to get mumps, measles and rubella (still called German measles in them days); the MMR vaccine, which whatever anyone tells you immunises at high rates against all three for life – the immune system is truly amazing – was not widely introduced until the 1980s.

I caught all four viruses as a child, though in each case incredibly mildly (*my* immune system is truly amazing). My battle with chickenpox was limited to a single spot, albeit a very bad one on my abdomen. I also got away with barely noticeable cases of mumps and both types of measles, though my sister wasn't so lucky. Mum had a zero-tolerance policy towards sick days and sent her to school when she was in the early stages of measles. Even when school sent her back home due to a suspicious-looking red rash and a spot of vomiting, my mum was still sceptical.

Because of MMR, hardly anybody has the luxury of being sent home from school with measles any more, though many parents still cling to the unscientific belief that the vaccine is potentially harmful. And so all three viruses are still in circulation, preying on the vulnerable children whose parents would prefer them to get a life-threatening disease rather than a life-saving medicine. (It is always worth pointing out that the charlatan who started the anti-MMR movement, the struck-off doctor formerly known as Dr Andrew Wakefield, was not just wrong, but also mendacious. His research paper claiming a spurious link between MMR and autism was not just retracted, it was exposed as a deliberate fraud, which led to him being struck off the UK General Medical Council's register of official medical practitioners.)

Despite its reputation as a routine childhood infection, measles is decidedly not a minor disease. A quarter of people who get it need hospital treatment and up to one in 500 die from it. So we will leave that there. Mumps, too, is no trivial matter as it can cause infertility in men. Rubella is generally mild; about half of people who get it have no symptoms and the rest almost all get better of their own accord in a few days – hence its other alternative name, three-day measles. It was called German measles because its distinctness from regular measles was first recognised and promoted by German doctors. It is arguably the most generic of the many mild rash-causing infections, with a course that goes something like this: feel a bit shit, get a rash, feel better. Scarlet fever is another variation on this theme, though in its early stages it can also afflict the tongue, making it look uncannily like a strawberry (see page 154). Another is erythema infectiosum, which is widely known by its common name 'slapped cheek disease', as the main symptom is a vivid red rash on the face. It is a shame that it does not also affect the buttocks. Slapped arse disease!

Both my boys had the MMR jab and both are just fine. Neither got the chickenpox vaccine, however, because it is not on the UK's roster of routine childhood vaccinations. Several chickenpox vaccines exist and work very well, but they ain't worth the money. For one thing, chickenpox rarely requires medical treatment so immunising against it is a net drain on public finances. More importantly, having the virus circulating in the population is, on balance, good for both the public's health and its finances, as older adults who come into contact with it are less likely to get shingles, which costs a fortune to treat. Shingles – also called zoster – is caused by the same virus as chickenpox, but we will return to that.

The virus is called varicella-zoster virus (VZV; varicella is an alternative name for chickenpox denoting that it is a diminutive version of the dreaded smallpox, or variola). It is a highly contagious airborne virus, spread largely by the coughs and sneezes that are an early symptom of the disease, but also by touching the distinctive skin blisters. The incubation period is ten to twenty-one days; people become infectious a couple of days before the rash appears and remain so until every blister has crusted over, which usually starts around day four but can take a week or more to complete.

The classic chickenpox rash starts out as small red blotches that then fill with fluid and become itchy blisters up to a centimetre across. Their appearance at this stage has romantically been described as 'a dewdrop on a rose petal', but that does not last long. A few days later they might be described as 'a scab on a slice of meat' as they burst and crust over. That, however, may not be the end of it. The spots can come in waves and as one batch is crusting over, another can just be getting going.

The severity of the blistering varies a lot, from my solo effort to 500 or more. Blisters in close proximity can merge, forming superblisters. They can damage the skin badly enough to leave scars called pockmarks, or poxmarks (both words are derived from *pocc*, the Old English word for 'blister'). Get out your tiny violins, as my lonesome spot left a really big scar that could almost have been mistaken for a second belly button.

Because of the rash, chickenpox is classified as an 'exanthemic' disease, meaning it causes an exanthem, or extensive rash, on the outsides of humans. Rashes are an extremely common symptom of infectious diseases, but arise for many different reasons (see page 66).

In the case of chickenpox, the rash is a cunning part of the virus's plan to infect as many people as possible. The virus makes a beeline for the skin via the bloodstream, which it invades via the lymphatic system after gaining entry through the tonsils. When a virus particle reaches its target, it invades a cell and starts replicating, eventually bursting the cell so its replicons can infect others around it. The burst cell dies and its contents are disgorged; as the infection burns through skin cells in an ever-increasing circle, these cellular remains, plus pus and tissue fluid, accumulate under the epidermis and form the circular blister. Or dew drop, if you insist.

The 'dew' in the blister is a toxic reservoir of highly infectious virus; evolution, being brutish and uncaring, has selected them to be maddeningly itchy so the poxy person scratches and bursts them, thus giving the virus further opportunity to spread itself. Successfully so; the R_0 number of chickenpox – the average number of people that an infected person infects – is around eight. Somebody who is not immune has a 90 per cent chance of catching it from an infected housemate.

The immune system eventually defeats the infection, but often fails to mop it up completely. The surviving viruses go into hiding in nerve cells, storing up trouble for later. A very small proportion of cases progress to severe illness due to complications including pneumonia and inflammation of the brain, and there are a handful of recorded fatalities. Severe illness and death are more common in adults; adults are twenty-five times more likely than children to die from chickenpox. Exactly why adults are hit harder is not known, but similar disparities have been seen with other infectious diseases.

For this reason, parents of young children in places where vaccination is not routine are understandably keen to get it over and done with. When my sons were little, I discovered the existence of the chickenpox party, where parents send their kids round to an infected friend's house in an attempt to get them to catch the disease. I never had the chance to attend such a wonderful occasion. My sons caught it in the wild. We did not throw a party.

A single encounter with the virus (or vaccine) is usually enough for the human immune system to form a long-term memory of it, conferring lifelong immunity to the disease. But that does not prevent reinfection: people who have had chickenpox can still catch the virus, but their virus-primed immune system quashes it before it can make them ill.

Because of this, chickenpox is considered an ongoing and endless pandemic. If only all pandemic viruses were so benign . . .

The word 'pox' is a catch-all term for infectious diseases that produce pustules or eruptions on the skin. The chicken variety is by far the most common human pox, which is somewhat ironic as it is not caused by a pox virus. VZV is actually a herpes virus.

Many non-human animals are plagued by pox viruses, including monkeys, mice, pigs, sheep, goats and squirrels. Our own specialist pox virus, *Variola*, which causes smallpox, was eradicated in the wild in 1977. Humans can catch monkey and cowpox, and chimps and gorillas can catch chickenpox. Chickens also get the pox, but not chickenpox. Theirs is called fowlpox.

The origin of the name 'chickenpox' is obscure. It may be a bastardisation of 'itching pox', or be derived from the fact that children were affectionately known as chickens. Some more far-fetched explanations are that the blisters resemble chickpeas, or look like the pecks of a chicken. Maybe we should rename it 'dewdrop-on-a-rose-petalpox'.

In about 30 per cent of older people who had chickenpox in their youth, the hunkered-down virus reactivates and bursts out of its nerve cell refuge, triggering an outbreak of shingles. Also known as herpes zoster, the main symptom is a painful rash that blisters up and can last for weeks. It can also develop into a serious pain syndrome called post-herpetic neuralgia. The rash often occurs around the waist, hence the names: shingles is derived from *cingulum*, which is Latin for 'girdle', and *zoster* means 'belt' in Greek. Shingles is not a minor illness; in Britain the NHS spends a fortune treating it and offers people over seventy a vaccine. People with shingles can infect those who have not had the virus and give them chickenpox, starting the cycle all over again. My ex-flatmate and I are now approaching shingles territory; we are still friends. I bet he gets it way worse than me.

Glandular fever

If chickenpox is the quintessential childhood infection, then mononucleosis is the quintessential teenage one. It is caused by a virus that is spread via saliva, hence its nickname, 'the kissing disease'. Contrary to popular belief, it is not especially contagious but a prolonged round of tonsil hockey with an infected person is a fairly reliable way of catching it. There is no need for parents to arrange mono parties; they usually organise themselves.

When I was of snogging age, mono was still called glandular fever, which is a perfectly serviceable name for a disease whose symptoms include a fever and swollen 'glands' (which are not glands but lymph nodes, see page 233). Mono – or infectious mononucleosis to give it its official title – is more commonly used in the US, and may thus seem like an unnecessary neologism. But as happens so often when speakers of British English moan about vulgar Americanisms, mono actually takes precedence. The name was coined in the US in 1920, which is before the term glandular fever had made its way from German (*Drüsenfieber*) into English.

Mononucleosis is any condition that leads to a higher-than-normal count of a type of white blood cell called monocytes, which is how the disease was confirmed for years until a better, antibody-based assay was invented.

Despite its reputation as a teenage disease, many people get infected as children and show no or only very mild symptoms. People who don't catch it as children usually get it soon after, once the snogging starts. About 90 per cent of people worldwide have had it before their thirtieth birthday.

I was diagnosed with it around fourteen, which is incontrovertible proof that kissing is not the only way to catch it. It is also transmitted by coughs and sneezes, and by sharing cups or cutlery. Snogging is a no-no after diagnosis, but by then the damage has usually been done. The incubation period is four to six weeks and a carrier is infectious for much of this period. Doctors also advise against drinking alcohol as the virus can inflame the liver. As Adam Ant almost sang, can't drink, can't snog, what can you do?

In about 90 per cent of cases, mono is caused by a type of herpes virus called Epstein-Barr virus (EBV). But a handful of other viruses cause identical symptoms. The most common of these is another herpes virus, human cytomegalovirus (CMV).

The classic symptoms of mono in teenagers are fever and swollen lymph nodes, plus a sore throat. Often a *very* sore throat: the virus can infect both the tonsils and the pharynx, or back of the throat, badly enough to make them ooze pus and make swallowing very painful. Headaches and nausea and vomiting are not unusual. These acute symptoms usually clear up in a couple of weeks but feelings of general malaise and fatigue can linger for weeks or even months. There is no vaccine and no cure, and unlike many viral infections once we have had it, the virus sticks around in our bodies for life. We seem to reach a truce with it: the immune system tolerates it as long as it doesn't start fomenting further trouble. The symptoms eventually fade away, and you cannot get it twice. Which is a decent excuse for a teenage rampage.

Cold sores

A dog is for life, not just for Christmas. And so is a cold sore. If you get one of these painful little blisters, probably by kissing somebody who also has one, possibly at a drunken Christmas party, you have formed at least one lifelong relationship. The sore will go away eventually but the virus that causes it will not. It retreats into nerve cells and goes dormant, but may periodically re-animate for a repeat performance.

That virus is called herpes simplex 1, and is among the commonest pathogens of humans. Around two-thirds of people worldwide carry it, which if anything is surprisingly low given how common, infectious and easily spread it is. The usual way of catching it is intimate oral-to-oral contact, or kissing. Maybe the reason it isn't higher is that people with weeping or crusty lesions on or near their lips don't look all that kissable.

A cold sore usually starts as a burning or tingling sensation in a localised area. For experienced users, this is a signal that it is time to stock up on cold sore cream, because in twelve to forty-eight hours the area will probably erupt one or more fluid-filled blisters, which are where the virus is replicating inside skin cells and bursting them open to complete its not-quite-life cycle. A day or two later, the blisters burst to leave open sores, which then crust over and heal. This sequence takes around fourteen days from start to finish and the area is contagious throughout, including the tingly stage and particularly in the open-sore one. Some carriers become infectious from time to time even though they have no symptoms. So you don't have to drop your usual standards to catch a cold sore.

You also don't have to have kissed a carrier recently to develop a debut sore. Many years can elapse between catching the virus and it bursting onto the scene. This is a useful thing to know if you have a cold sore and a suspicious romantic partner.

First-time outbreaks are sometimes also accompanied by mild flu-like symptoms. But subsequent ones are very localised to the places where the virus can hide.

Cold sores do not always recur – about two-thirds of people who develop one never get another – but when they do, they always hit the same spot. These secondary outbreaks can strike three or more times a year but tend to be milder than the first, because the immune system is primed to deal with the virus. They also become less frequent with age, for the same reason.

Exactly what triggers the virus to reactivate is not known, but some frequent fliers notice obvious triggers. Sunshine is one. For some reason, ultraviolet light is a mild immunosuppressant of the skin, which may compromise the immune system's ability to keep the virus in check. Fatigue and stress also negatively impact the immune system and are known to reactivate latent cold sores. So can colds and other respiratory-tract infections, hence the name 'cold sore'. They are also known as fever blisters.

Cold sore creams, some containing anti-viral drugs, are quite effective at helping the sores to heal quickly but won't prevent them. Research on a vaccine has been ongoing for around a century, thus far without success.

The virus can cause lesions on other parts of the body too, especially the fingers. These painful lesions are essentially cold sores, though they go by the archaic-sounding name of herpetic whitlows. A whitlow is a painful lesion on the fingertip; the name is of Germanic origin and means 'white crack'. Herpetic whitlows are red sores, but we will let it go.

The herpes simplex 1 virus can also infect the genitals, but we won't go there. Ditto the closely related herpes simplex 2 virus, which is an occasional cause of oral cold sores but prefers the genitals.

HSV1 and 2 are members of a large virus family, the Herpesviridae, which are an endless scourge of humanity. The name is derived from the Greek for 'creep', which is entirely appropriate. Not only do they cause cold sores and genital herpes, they are also responsible for chickenpox and shingles (see page 242), glandular fever (see page 248) and various low-level flu-like infections such as cytomegalovirus, which chronically infects pretty much everybody worldwide and has been inconclusively linked to all sorts of grumbling health problems. You may not like the idea that you have herpes, but you probably do. For life.

Fungus the bogeyman

I'm not much of an athlete these days, but I do have very athletic feet. By which I mean they are infected with a fungus that evidently finds the warm and moist areas between my toes very much to its liking.

I don't know exactly what kind of fungus it is: there are about forty species that make a living by eating human skin. Collectively known as dermatophytes – from the Greek for 'skin plant' – they also infect other parts of the body, causing ringworm, jock itch, scalp itch, nail infections, a fungal infection of the facial hair follicles called barber's itch, and more. Wherever there's some skin to munch, a fungus will try to eat it for lunch.

In the pantheon of pathogenic microorganisms, fungi really are the least of our worries. Compared with bacteria and viruses, they are neither very dangerous nor hard to cure. They tend to cause only superficial infections of the skin and are easy to eradicate. But not before they have inflicted itchy, flaky, painful and sometimes broken skin on their victims. As the old joke goes, these fungi are not fun guys to be with.

The fungi that infest our skin are mostly moulds, which produce networks of filaments like the black mould that grows on old food. They eat keratin, a fibrous protein that toughens the skin and also forms hair and nails. Rhino horn is made almost entirely of keratin, which proves that people who eat it to improve their sex lives are little better than the parasites growing between my toes.

The formal medical name for a fungal infection of the skin is tinea, which is the Latin word for any sort of beetle grub that devours organic material such as paper or wool. Tineas are further categorised according to location on the body, so foot fungus is called tinea pedis, inner-thigh fungus tinea cruris, scalp fungus tinea capitis, and so on.

Athlete's foot is very common – about 15 per cent of people have it at any one time, most of them men because they have sweatier feet. A further 5 per cent have a tinea somewhere else on their body.

Tineas of all kinds are picked up through contact with other infected people or animals – cats and dogs can get ringworm too and will pass it on to their humans.

Athlete's foot is especially infectious as you don't have to play footsie with someone to catch it. If somebody who has athlete's foot walks barefoot across a floor they can shed fungal spores that will readily take up residence on other passing feet. That is especially problematic in warm and moist environments where people often remove their shoes and socks, such as the changing rooms at swimming pools and gyms. Hence the name.

Once the fungus has a toehold (often literally), it can be transferred to other parts of the body by, say, itching the itchy skin between toes and then scratching your crotch.

Until quite recently almost nobody had fungus foot, and infections at the other end of the body were much more of a problem. In the early 1800s, ringworm of the scalp, commonly known as scald-head, spread like wildfire through the slums and newly established state schools of Britain's booming cities. It was considered a disease of the poor and unwashed, which is why in 1835 the country was scandalised by an outbreak at one of London's most prestigious private schools, Christ's Hospital.

Ringworm is not caused by a worm. It probably got its common name from the mistaken belief that it was caused by a skin-chomping beetle grub, plus the fact that it typically presents as a ring of red rash. Its true origin was established not long after the outbreak at the school, which helped –

along with an aggressive and largely successful public health campaign – to eradicate it.

Although ringworm has been known for centuries, athlete's foot was a rare condition until quite recently. The first medical description was published in 1908 by Arthur Whitfield, a skin specialist at King's College in London. A patient was referred to him with chronic inflammation and cracking of the skin on his feet. The man had been diagnosed with eczema (see page 68), but Whitfield begged to differ. He took a skin sample from between the patient's toes – which he vividly described as being 'sodden' – examined it under a microscope and saw what was unmistakeably a fungus known to cause ringworm. He diagnosed ringworm of the foot and prescribed the standard fungicidal treatment at the time, a highly toxic compound called perchloride of mercury. It didn't work, and the patient stopped coming. But he nevertheless went down in medical history as the first confirmed case of athlete's foot.

It wasn't called that at the time, of course. The name appears to have originated in the US in the 1920s during an epidemic of ringworm of the foot fuelled by the growth in popularity of swimming pools, sports clubs, vigorous sweaty exercise and, paradoxically, foot hygiene. Frequent washing and exfoliating moisturise and soften the skin and make it easier for the fungus to break in. The name was eagerly adopted by the leisured middle classes who wanted to avoid the stigma of ringworm, which was still considered a scourge of the filthy urban poor.

Athlete's foot is also exacerbated by wearing socks and shoes – especially those made from non-breathable synthetic materials – which create a very cosy environment for fungi. In places where people habitually go barefoot, athlete's foot remains rare.

The modern vice of socks can also make treating athlete's foot a cycle of triumph and disaster as hard-to-kill fungal spores lodge in the fabric and constantly reinfect the toes. Bleach and a hot wash (of socks, not toes) can kill them. Shoes can also harbour the fungus and are harder to decontaminate. Sometimes the only option is to chuck them. People with chronic athlete's foot are advised not to wear the same pair of shoes for more than two days in a row, and to go barefoot at every opportunity.

Dermatophyte infections can be itchy and sometimes painful, causing the skin to crack, bleed and even blister. But they are easily wiped out using anti-fungal creams, powders, nail varnishes and sprays. More persistent infections, such as of the nail bed, may require antifungal tablets to shift them.

Dermatophytes are not our only fungal bogeymen. Some single-celled yeasts have also developed a taste for human skin and hair. The commonest is *Candida*, which thrives in warm, moist areas such as the mouth and genitals; infections are commonly called thrush because the yeast grows in white patches that resemble the breast of the garden bird. Another yeast called *Trichosporon* can grow in hair and cause a dandruff-like condition called white piedra. *Piedra* is Spanish for 'stone'. There is also black piedra, caused by a different fungus, characterised by small dark nodules on the hair shaft. Which just goes to show that there is no place on the human body where, given half a chance, a fungus of some kind won't gladly take up residence.

UTIs

One of my favourite jokes about anatomy (admittedly not an especially competitive category) goes something like this. Three engineers are arguing about what kind of engineer evolution is. The electrical engineer says electrical, because of the exquisite wiring of the nervous system. The chemical engineer says chemical, because metabolism is so amazing. Get outta here, says the civil engineer. Only a civil engineer would run a waste pipe through a recreational area.

There's nothing especially interesting, let alone amusing, to say about urinary tract infections. If it hurts when you pee, and/or if your pee is cloudy or smelly, and/or if you need to pee more often or more urgently than usual, chances are you have a UTI. That might mean an infection of the urethra or bladder (collectively called cystitis), or the kidneys. They are usually caused by bacteria and can be cleared out with antibiotics. Sometimes they clear up on their own, often they don't. Go see a doctor. And try not to use the area for recreation until the waste pipes are sorted.

Hayfever

I always know when spring is in the air, and it really gets up my nose. Some time in mid-February – not exactly a spring-like month in Britain, but the worst is behind us by then – my eyes and nose suddenly start to itch like mad. They torment me for about ten days then stop. I presume it is an allergic reaction to some sort of airborne pollen. In other words, allergic rhinitis, or hayfever.

Like all allergies, hayfever is an inappropriate immune response to something that ought not to bother it. As well as pollen from trees, grasses and weeds, it can be triggered by mould, dust, fungal spores and animal dander. When these are inhaled and settle on the moist lining of the nose and mouth, they come into contact with frontline immune cells called mast cells. These are supposed to repel actual invaders such as bacteria. But in people whose immune systems have, for reasons still unknown, gone a bit awry, they overreact. This causes the cells to disgorge a potent inflammatory com-pound called histamine. The result is floods of mucus to flush out the 'invader', leading to violent and slobbery sneezing and itchy inflammation. Mast cells are also found in the lining of the eyelids.

Britain may no longer be a global power, but it is the undisputed hayfever champion of the world with a preva-lence of about 30 per cent and rising. That is double the global average, which is also rising. Why it is going up we do not know.

Hayfever takes its name from its historical association with the haying season, when farmers cut grasses to lay down for winter fodder and probably sent plumes of pollen into the air. It was officially recognised in 1819 when a London doctor called John Bostock described his own symptoms in one of the journals of the Royal Society of Medicine. He described it as a rare condition.

Hayfever is not specific to hay or the summer; almost any pollen from any wind-pollinated plant can trigger it, at almost any time of year. There are hundreds of known allergenic pollens and many people are allergic to two or more, meaning that some people's hayfever season can last for months.

The immune response is typically triggered once the pollen count reaches fifty, which means there are fifty grains of pollen per cubic metre of air. A single ragweed plant – a major cause of hayfever – can release 2.5 billion pollen grains a day.

I have no idea exactly what triggers my February fever and long ago gave up trying to find out. There are so many possible suspects, and knowing which one is guilty would not bring any relief. Whatever it is, I cannot avoid it, indoors or out. And in any case hayfever is managed the same way whatever the cause, with antihistamines and other over-the-counter remedies.

Before I have bought my supply (I never remember to do it in advance), I am almost unable to resist rubbing my itchy eyes. But this just grinds the allergen deeper in and spreads it around to yet more over-eager mast cells. I rediscover this fact every February.

Insect bites

A few days before I wrote this piece, I was attacked by a predator. It sneaked up, ate some of me, and then vanished into the twilight. I didn't even realise it had attacked me until the next morning, when I woke up with bite marks all over my legs.

We humans don't tend to think of ourselves as prey, but we are. Admittedly the risks are much lower than they once were – our ancestors on the African savannah endured high levels of predation from eighteen or so species of large carnivorous mammal that were around at the time. But there are still plenty of species that make a living from eating humans, though thankfully not whole ones any more.

Spoiler alert: this is the longest section in the book, because there are an awful lot of people-eating monsters to write about.

I suspect the monster that attacked me in my own back garden over an early-evening beer was a banded house mosquito (*Culiseta annulata*), the largest and commonest species of mosquito in Britain. The females of this species are haematophagous, meaning blood-eating. But it could have been any one of thirty-three other species of mosquito found in Britain, including a recent invader from the Far East called the Asian tiger mosquito (*Aedes albopictus*).

Or maybe it was a horse fly, a midge, a gnat or a flea. All can cause the red, swollen and excruciatingly itchy welts that tormented me for days afterwards. You generally can't tell after the fact what sucked some of your blood. But I can take comfort from the fact that it wasn't a tick, of which more later.

Many other arthropods can also deliver a nasty bite, though for self-defence rather than dinner. That includes ants, spiders and the peaceful-sounding but actually quite aggressive flower bugs. And if they don't get you, maybe the ladybirds will; they can give quite a nip if provoked. So don't go around provoking ladybirds.

All of these bites are generally harmless and easily treated, though they can occasionally turn very nasty. And of course in some countries mosquitoes and other blood-sucking insects are vectors of serious diseases including malaria, yellow fever, dengue, zika and West Nile. By some estimates, mosquito-borne diseases have killed half the people who ever lived, making them by far the deadliest predator of humans. I can count myself lucky that malaria was eliminated from Britain more than 100 years ago and if it does make a come-back due to climate change, it probably won't happen until the 2050s, by which time I will probably have joined the half of humanity who died of something else.

All told, there are around 3,500 species of mosquito. Despite their fearsome reputation, the vast majority are peace-loving vegetarians, deploying their elongated mouth-parts to sip at plant sap, nectar and the honeydew produced by aphids. But in many species the females – the bloodsuck-ers are always female – are also capable of piercing the skin of much larger animals and drinking their blood. A recent analysis concluded that this evolved as a back-up plan to stay hydrated during intense dry seasons, but some species evidently developed a taste for the hard stuff and never went back.

Mosquitoes can guzzle up to three times their own body-weight in blood, and will even excrete the liquid part of blood from their anus while still drinking in order to gorge on the solid bits. To something as small as a mosquito, drinking blood must be rather like sucking baked beans through a tube.

Some species are fussy about their prey, but others will attack pretty much anything that moves. Mosquitoes are known to bite mammals, birds, reptiles and even fish. Some will even suck the blood of other insects.

They have plagued humanity for millennia; some Egyptian curses include mosquito hieroglyphs and tests on mummies have found high levels of the malaria parasite *Plasmodium falciparum*. In the fifth century BC, the Greek historian Herodotus reported that the builders of the pyramids (already ancient history by then) were fed large amounts of leeks, onions and radishes to ward off mosquitoes. There is some evidence that people who eat a lot of garlic are less troubled by mosquitoes, presumably because the little buggers don't like the smell or taste.

Blood-sucking female mosquitoes need blood to complete their life cycle as it contains proteins and fats that are required for egg maturation. A female will typically eat once, then lay. It is often said that she then dies, her work done. But this is a myth. After laying one batch of eggs a female is often back in the market for a mate, and another bloody meal.

When a bloodthirsty female mosquito lands on your skin, she rarely dives straight in but first prods around with her proboscis feeling for a suitable spot. If you are lucky your itch sensors will detect her before she finds one and cause you to swat her away (see page 76).

But if not, once the mosquito has located a promising watering hole she painlessly pierces the skin with her needle-like mouthparts and pushes through until she hits a blood vessel. She has no need to suck; blood is pressurised and flows passively through the tubular mouthparts (one of my other favourite Far Side cartoons by Gary Larson is a grossly distended feeding mosquito being shouted at by another: 'Pull out, Betty! You've hit an artery'). But she does need to blow, in order to inject saliva into the vessel to keep the blood flowing.

The saliva typically contains proteins designed to hijack the victim's biology: vasodilators to open up the blood vessel and anticoagulants to stop clots from gumming up the mouthparts. It is these rather than the puncture wound that cause us so much aggravation. Once the mosquito is gorged, she withdraws her proboscis and buzzes off. If you happen to mete out lethal punishment to a mozzie after she has eaten, your wall or ceiling will be smeared with human blood, quite possibly your own.

Even before the mosquito withdraws, the foreign proteins in her saliva set alarm bells ringing in the immune system. The first responders are histamines, inflammatory compounds released by immune cells in the skin in response to foreign proteins. Histamines increase the permeability of capillaries, allowing white blood cells to squeeze out and hunt down the invaders. One side effect of this is swelling and itchiness, which can sometimes progress to a large fluid-filled blister.

The itch from a mosquito bite can last for several days, and scratching it only makes it worse because it stimulates the release of yet more histamines. Relief can be found in the many antihistamine and corticosteroid creams and ointments that can be bought over the counter; ditto ammonia solutions. But the traditional home remedies of vinegar and bicarbonate of soda are useless.

You can also buy zappers that deliver a small electric shock to the site of a bite. They look like mini-tasers with two pointy electrodes about half a centimetre apart, which deliver a short high-voltage but low-current discharge at the click of a button. The theory behind them is that the electric shock warms the area between the electrodes and inhibits histamine release. Whether or not this is true, a test carried out by the FDA found that they really do reduce itching.[43]

Which I'm glad about, because my wife spends a fortune on them. One year we went on holiday to a charming but mozzie-infested region of Italy, and the soundtrack of the summer was the constant click-click-click of a Zap-It!

Mosquito Insect Bite Relief Device. Each zapper can supposedly treat 1,000 bites at five to ten zaps per bite before running out of zap. I swear she and her brother were zapping their way through that every day.

To be fair, she is a mosquito magnet. It is common knowledge that some people get bitten more than others and, unlike most pieces of common knowledge, this one is true.

In the 1970s, researchers at the London School of Hygiene and Tropical Medicine deliberately exposed 162 volunteers to *Anopheles gambiae* mosquitoes, the most virulent vector of malaria in sub-Saharan Africa.[44] The volunteers had to sit for ten minutes in dim red light with their arm exposed while bloodthirsty mozzies buzzed around them. The researchers counted how many 'blood meals' each volunteer provided, then killed the mosquitoes and tested what blood group the ingested blood belonged to. They found that humans belonging to the type-O blood group were significantly more attractive to the mozzies. My wife is type-O. I am type-A, so I like to be with her when mosquitoes are about.

Further research has found exactly the same preference in other species of mosquito. Exactly why they prefer type-O blood is not known, though it seems they can smell it on us. Some people are known to secrete markers of their blood-type onto their skin, and O-types who do so are even more attractive to mosquitoes.

Some mosquito species can also smell compounds found in sweat and exhaled breath, including carbon dioxide, and will follow an airborne trail of them to land themselves a meal. They are also heat-seeking and are more strongly attracted to people who have been drinking alcohol. So hot, sweaty, heavy-breathing drunks are also mosquito magnets. I am not suggesting for a moment that my wife is any of those things. She would probably say I am all of them.

The link between alcohol consumption and mozzie bites raises an intriguing question, perhaps best articulated by the sozzled *Ab Fab* character Patsy: 'The last mosquito that bit me had to check into the Betty Ford Clinic.' Whether mosquitoes become intoxicated by drinking the blood of drunk people is not known, but if anybody wants to run a study on that, I am volunteering.

There is also variation in the immune response to mosquito bites, largely dependent on previous exposure. This further explains why some people seem more prone to bites than others. They don't necessarily get bitten more, but their response to bites is more extreme.

In 1946, entomologist Kenneth Mellanby of the London School of Hygiene and Tropical Medicine investigated this phenomenon.[45] He recruited twenty-five volunteers who had never been outside of Britain and subjected them to repeated attacks by the tropical mosquito *Aedes aegypti*. He noted a stereotypical pattern of responses. The first time they were bitten, the volunteers had no immediate reaction but after twenty-four hours they all had itchy red lumps at the bite sites. After a month of being repeatedly bitten, their responses had become more extreme. As soon as they were bitten, they came out in welts that lasted for about two hours, and also got the itchy red lumps after twenty-four hours. After another month, however, though the welts still appeared, the delayed reaction had vanished. And eventually, after thousands of bites, they no longer had a reaction at all. Mellanby saw the same pattern with other species of mosquito. So if you have a bad reaction to mosquito bites, take comfort that you will eventually become immune.

There is also the question of whether mosquitoes prefer to bite certain parts of the body. Itchy bites certainly seem to be more common on the ankles, feet, face and neck. That may be because mosquito attractors such as breath and sweat are more concentrated in those regions. But it may also be because those areas are less padded by fat and muscle, so the itch itches worse.

If mosquitoes are the pickpockets of the bloodsucker world, horseflies are the smash-and-grab merchants. They too mostly eat veggie food but the females need a blood meal to produce eggs. But instead of surgically piercing the skin with a delicate proboscis they rake at it with dagger-like projections and then slurp up the blood that oozes out. This butchery often alerts the victim to the attack and the horsefly gets a slap, meaning they may have to visit several large animals to obtain a bellyful. Their saliva contains anticoagulants that raise an immune response, but their slobbery mouthparts are also often contaminated with blood and other gubbins from previous unsuccessful attacks. The bites they leave behind are consequently sorer, itchier and longer-lasting than mozzie bites, and often get infected. But again they can almost always be treated with over-the-counter bite creams and antiseptics.

Gnats and midges – which are not well-defined taxonomic groups but rather colloquial terms for any number of small blood-sucking flies including sandflies and blackflies – are essentially mini-horseflies, employing a similar slash-and-slurp feeding technique but on smaller scales. They are often tiny, hence the nickname no-see-ums. But their bites are worse than their buzz, and can be as painful and itchy as a mosquito bite.

All of these bitey little bastards can be repelled by covering up and wearing insect repellent. The synthetic jungle juice diethyltoluamide (DEET), which was developed by the US military for soldiers fighting jungle warfare, is the most effective. But more natural incense-like mosquito coils and citronella candles, which are burned to produce an insect-repellent smokescreen, have been shown to be better than nothing.

Fleas use a slightly different method of attack. Their mouthparts feature a pair of barbs that slice the skin and then jack open the wound so that a central proboscis can be inserted to suck up the blood. They also inject an anticoagulant which triggers an immune response and leads to red, itchy bites. Flea bites are almost invariably inflicted by fleas from household pets, which prefer cats and dogs but will eat human blood if hungry; there is a species of flea that prefers human company (though all fleas are promiscuous to some extent) but it is vanishingly rare these days.

Ticks are another bitey menace. They are mites that lurk in long grass, fling themselves onto passing animals, find a suitable spot for lunch and dig in. Like fleas they first slice a hole in the skin, then insert a specialised feeding tube. In ticks this is called a hypostome, a barbed structure not unlike a rawlplug with backward-pointing projections that stop it from being pulled out. The tick also secretes a sort of glue. Together these firmly anchor the tick in place so it can settle in and eat its fill, which is a lot. A tick can feed continuously for several days and consume around 500 times its own bodyweight in blood. Mr Creosote eat your heart out.

Once full, the tick dissolves the glue, withdraws its hypostome and drops off the host. It accomplishes its feat of endurance and concealment by injecting anti-inflammatory proteins called, deliciously, evasins into the wound, which stop the bite from swelling and itching – at least while the tick is attached. Once it has detached, the bite can become swollen, itchy and bruised or even blistered. Tick bites are not to be taken lightly, as ticks carry the potentially serious bacterial infection Lyme disease. If you discover a bite that is surrounded by a circular red rash, sometimes with a halo of rash around it like the bullseye on a dartboard, go to the doctor.

And if you catch a tick in the act of lunching, resist the temptation to yank it off. You will probably decapitate it and leave the head and mouthparts embedded. Gently pull it out using tweezers (if you still decapitate it the mouthparts can usually be tweezed out separately, but if not leave it alone and your immune system will deal with it). Then exact your revenge. The US Centers for Disease Control and Prevention recommends dropping ticks into alcohol, wrapping them in tape or flushing them down the toilet. It warns that the old-fashioned method of burning a tick off with the tip of a lit cigarette does not work. It can just cause the tick to regurgitate all the blood back into the wound and increase the odds of getting an infection.

Similar to ticks are another group of parasitic mites commonly called chiggers or harvest mites. They also lurk in the undergrowth and leap onto passing animals, but rather than sucking blood they chomp skin. Once they have a firm grip, they spew digestive enzymes which erode a hole in the skin, from which the chigger then feeds. Their 'bites' can become red, itchy and inflamed.

Mere mention of the word 'chigger' is enough to make me shudder. When I was ten, I spent a long and glorious summer living in New Mexico with my mum, dad and sister. My dad was there for work (yes, bracken grows there); we were there for fun, of which we had lots. The local kids were morbidly obsessed with chigger bites, which they said would swell and swell until they burst and disgorged thousands of baby chiggers. They all claimed to know somebody who knew somebody that this had happened to. It was also said to be a hazard of spider bites. I was always getting bitten by things – it was 1980 and insect repellent was an unknown substance to English people – and feared the worst. It never happened, because it is an urban myth. Chiggers are baby mites anyway – the larval stage is the skin-munching time of their life cycle – and they do not lay eggs at all, let alone in their feeding holes. Spiders do not either; in fact, there are zero species of spider that feed directly on human flesh, though plenty that will give you a nasty bite.

However, as with many urban myths, the baby chigger one does have a passing acquaintance with the truth. Some flies lay their eggs in or near open wounds and their larvae, also known as maggots, develop under the skin. Others cunningly lay their eggs on the mouthparts of mosquitoes and other biting insects and get them to do their dirty work for them. Maggot invasions of the nasal passages and ear canals are also possible. Fortunately, this rare and disgusting condition, called myiasis, is largely confined to the tropics, though is not unknown in the US. So it is possible that my New Mexican playmates really did know somebody who knew somebody that this had happened to. I think I'm safe in my own back garden.

But something I'm decidedly not safe from is yet another insect that likes to lurk around humans and bite chunks out of them: the bedbug. Actually two species of insect, *Cimex lectularius* and *Cimex hemipterus*, they take up residence in bedding, mattresses, chairs, sofas and under picture frames and loose wallpaper. Like mini vampires, they come out at night and suck blood, often from the neck.

Bedbugs are quite big – about 5 millimetres long – reddish-brown in colour and look a bit like small, flattened cockroaches. They shit the bed, so a tell-tale sign that they have been around is small brown spots on your sheets. Plus small red spots on the neck, arms, legs or another patch of skin that was exposed while asleep, fresh batches of which appear every morning. The bites can be sore and itchy and often appear in clusters or straight lines, as the bug likes to take several bites of the cherry. As with most insect bites, the itchiness is an immune response to the bedbug's anticoagulant and painkilling saliva, which it delivers via toothed mouthparts that it moves back and forth to saw through skin and draw blood. The bugs also emit a sweetish musty smell that has been likened to coriander seeds.

Bedbugs are less common than they once were, largely due to an all-out insecticide assault after the Second World War. The great chronicler of early-twentieth century poverty, George Orwell, often dwelt on the horrors of bugs. The various flophouses he stayed in in Paris and London were invariably crawling with them. 'Near the ceiling long lines of bugs marched all day like columns of soldiers,' he wrote of the not-very-charming Hôtel des Trois Moineaux in the Latin Quarter, 'and at night came down ravenously hungry, so that one had to get up every few hours and kill them.'

Bedbugs have evolved resistance to many insecticides and are staging a comeback. They thrive in warmth, so widespread use of central heating and climate change are also giving them a leg up. They often hitch a ride on public transport – trains, planes, buses and subways are a great pick-up spot for bugs, which we then take home to bed. Hotel rooms, Airbnbs and backpacker hostels are another source. People often return from their travels with a souvenir they did not bargain for.

Getting rid of bed bugs is not easy. Squish any that you see, which was how they were dealt with in Orwell's day. Wash infested bedding and clothes in a sixty-degree wash to boil them alive, or put them in the freezer to freeze them to death. Hoover thoroughly. If possible, switch beds for a couple of weeks to starve them, too. If that doesn't work, a visit from pest control may be in order.

Another parasitic lover of human bedding is *Sarcoptes scabiei*, microscopic mites that live most of their lives in hair follicles, where they feed and mate (yes, there are mites having sex in your hair follicles). Once impregnated, the females leave the follicles and start digging, burrowing into skin to lay eggs. Also known as the itch mite, the tunnels they excavate in the outer layer of skin become intensely itchy, a very common condition called scabies. The itch is caused by the tunnelling itself – which the mite carries out with her mouthparts and cutting tools on her front legs, like a microscopic tunnel-boring machine – and also an immune response to the mite and her eggs. The rash often starts between the fingers but can spread across the whole body, though rarely affects the head (maybe the mites are afraid of their distant and relatively monstrous cousins, lice – see page 273).

Scabies rashes are often linear or S-shaped because the mites tunnel determinedly in one direction. They are also digging their own graves; after laying a line of thirty or so eggs at a rate of one or two a day, the exhausted female expires.

If they are not red the burrows may appear silvery, which is the colour of mite eggs under the skin. When the eggs hatch the tiny mites dig their way out and seek out a hair follicle in which to feed, mature, have sex and start the whole ghastly process all over again.

Scabies is extremely infectious via skin-to-skin contact. It has nothing to do with poor hygiene. But it can be passed on during sex, so people with scabies are advised to abstain for the several days it takes to clear up. They are also advised to contact trace anyone they have had sex with in the previous eight weeks, as the early stages of a mite infestation (the having-sex-in-your-hair-follicles stage) can be entirely symptom-free.

If they do not die in a ditch of their own digging, itch mites are generally killed by chemical warfare. The standard treatment is a mite-killing cream or lotion that has to be smeared all over the body and left to do its mischief for several hours. These medications usually contain permethrin, an insecticide that is also used to kill lice and ward off mosquitoes. Mites are not insects – they are arachnids, so are more closely related to spiders – but are vulnerable to permethrin.

Scabies mites can also be passed to, and caught from, animals. In cats and dogs they are one of the main causes of mange. Don't pet a mangy dog or you might end up mangy yourself.

And that is the end of our adventures in bitey land. Night night, sleep tight, hope the bugs don't bite.

Lice

A friend of mine who shall remain nameless once caught crabs off a woman he shared a bed with in a squat. A few weeks later his nether regions were red, itchy and his pubic hair covered in small round blobs. He did not know what was wrong – his father was a man of the Church and he grew up in a straightlaced household, and the internet had not yet been invented – so went to a chemist and, with considerable embarrassment, described his troubles. She sold him some lotion and he went back to his family home to apply it. Job done, he took a shower. Seconds later his genital area was on fire and the more he rinsed the worse it got. Soon his mother was banging on the bathroom door shouting, 'Alexander, Alexander, are you all right in there?' (not his real name), like the bathroom scene from *Portnoy's Complaint* transferred to a small northern town.

After the fire died down and his mother had been placated, he re-read the instructions on the bottle. DO NOT WASH FOR AT LEAST EIGHT HOURS AFTER APPLICATION.

Crabs are a type of louse that have evolved to live in coarse human hair and drink human blood. That generally means pubic hair, but they will also colonise armpit hair, chest and back hair, facial hair and sometimes eyebrows and eyelashes. Head hair is out of bounds as it is too fine and densely packed for them.

Crabs are not crabs at all, but small wingless insects. They are obligate parasites – once described as predators that like their prey but couldn't eat a whole one – and die in a day or two if they are separated from their host, of both starvation and cold. If you catch crabs, that is the fate you will wish upon them. But separating them is easier said than done, as they tenaciously grip on to pubes with two large pairs of crab-like front claws.

Lice are the price we pay for being warm-blooded animals. There are around 5,000 species globally, and every known mammal and bird has one (or rarely two) that parasitises them, except for bats, pangolins, platypuses and echidnas. Humans are blessed with three, due to us offering three different habitats for them to live in: pubic hair, head hair and clothing.

Pubic lice are usually picked up by close contact, usually sexual, with an infested person. They can't jump. The most efficient way to transfer them is for two people to grind their pubic regions together for a while. Other close contact such as cuddling and kissing can also transfer them, as can – occasionally – simply sharing a bed with somebody. That is how my friend caught them. Poor guy: all the pain, none of the pleasure.

Crabs suck blood and the most noticeable symptom of an infestation is an itchy crotch, which is caused not by crabs crawling around but an immune response to their anticoagulant saliva which they inject through a barbed proboscis. The itch can be very itchy, especially at night when the crabs come out to feed. The area may also become inflamed and raw from scratching the infernal bites, which appear as small blue spots or tiny drops of blood on the skin.

The crabs themselves are quite small, no more than 1.8 millimetres long, and hard to see as they are brown and hence well camouflaged. They are also quite rare: a single pubic region can only sustain about twelve adult lice, though they may go a-wandering to find pastures new if there is a continuous route of hair up the navel.

More noticeable are their eggs, which they glue firmly to the shafts of pubic hairs and which, once hatched, turn white. Correct: the crabs are having sex in your pants. They are also crapping in your pants, depositing small dark droppings that accumulate in the gusset as a black powder.

They are easy to diagnose, but not to get rid of. Insecticides are the only real option but the little buggers have evolved resistance to many of the standard ones. Eradication requires two applications of pubic gloop about a week apart, the second one to wipe out any crabs that hatched after the first. It is advisable to wash clothes and bedding in hot water.

Crabs are not a vector for diseases but people sometimes find that they have picked up a sexually transmitted infection along with them. Infested people are advised to notify anyone they have had sexual contact with in the previous three months and get tested for STIs even if they do not have symptoms. Cue the blame game of who infested who.

Disgusted yet? There's more. The origin of pubic lice is, erm, interesting. Biologically they are distinct from the two other human-infesting species, head lice and clothes lice. So distinct, in fact, that they are classified in a different taxonomic group (the genus *Pthirus* as opposed to *Pediculus*). Head lice and clothes lice are clearly closely related to one another and also the lice that live on chimps. It seems that our ancestors were already lousy when the chimp and human lineages split about 6 million years ago.

But the closest living relative of the pubic louse is the louse that lives on . . . gorillas. Genetic evidence suggests that it crawled into our lineage about 4 million years ago. How that happened I will leave to your imagination. Maybe they just shared a bed.

Head lice are longer and slimmer than pubic lice and evolved to live in the denser, thinner head hair. They also drink our blood and glue their eggs to the bases of our hair shafts – these are the nits that are the signature of a head louse infestation. A full head of hair can sustain a population of up to twenty head lice. They are by far the most common species of human louse and can spread like wildfire through schools. Despite the stigma that is attached to them they do not prefer dirty hair. Most kids, even well-groomed ones, get them from time to time, and often pass them on to their parents and siblings. That is considered a public health good as it may mean we build up immune resistance to them and their much more problematic close relative the clothes louse.

Insecticidal shampoos and fine-toothed combs usually see them off, though like crabs they are increasingly resistant to the insecticides we try to kill them with. They do not transmit disease and don't cause much itching, though sometimes they can be felt wandering around on the scalp. They are essentially a cosmetic problem.

That is not true of clothes or body lice. They live inside clothing or bedclothes, clinging on to fibres and laying their eggs on them. They look exactly like head lice, though a bit longer. They do not live directly on the human body but will seek one out when hungry, which is about five times a day. For that reason, they prefer items of clothing that come into frequent contact with skin, such as underpants. An individual can be infested with thousands at once and get bitten to hell. This causes a skin disease called pediculosis corporis.

Thankfully, body lice are nowhere near as common as head lice because normal washing of clothes kills them, but infestations are known to break out in unsanitary places such as prisons, crowded slums and refugee camps. In some parts of the world they are vectors for some really nasty diseases including typhus and relapsing fever. During the First World War soldiers in the trenches were crawling with them and often went down with a louse-borne bacterial infection technically called Werner disease but commonly known as trench fever. Oh! What a lousy war.

Genetic comparison to head lice tells us that the two species diverged at least 83,000 years ago, which is considered to be excellent evidence that clothing had been invented by then.

Insect stings

As I mentioned earlier, it is a bad idea to provoke a ladybird lest you want a nasty nip. It is an even worse idea to provoke bees and wasps. They don't bite but they do sting, and will do so at the drop of a hat with much more painful results than anything a wussy ladybird can deliver. Their stings hurt not because they puncture the skin, but because they inject venom. These are complex mixtures of compounds that evolved to make us go away and not come back, which means inflicting pain.

I haven't been stung by a bee for years but I know somebody who has: my young nephew, who came running in from the back garden screaming, 'Fly, sore!' through his tears while pointing to something on his arm. It took us ages to work out what was wrong.

Poor little fella. Honeybee stings hurt, especially when you are yet to reach your second birthday. They are barbed and often get stubbornly stuck in the skin. The bee will try to extract its sting, but will usually fail and end up flying away without it, plus the venom sac and various bits of its insides. Unsurprisingly, this loss of vital organs is fatal, to the bee at least.

Even after the bee has buzzed off to expire, the detached venom sac continues to pump toxins into the wound and so removing the sting is priority number one. Doctors usually recommend scraping it off with a fingernail rather than pinching it out, as the latter can just squeeze more toxins into the wound. And the more toxins you get, the more painful the sting.

Wasp stings are not barbed so they can sting you repeatedly. Bumblebees also have smooth stings but they generally live up to their cuddly reputation and will only sting if severely provoked.

Some species of ant – which are closely related to bees and wasps in the order *Hymenoptera* – also have stingers at the end of their abdomens. The main pain-inducing ingredient of their venom is formic acid, named after the Latin word for ant, *formica*. As a rule, black ants don't sting but red ones do. Some ant stings are horrifically painful and seem unnecessarily sadistic. Fire ants, for example, grip their victim's skin with their powerful mandibles, plunge their sting into the skin, pull it out, rotate about their point of attachment and sting again, and so on until they complete a circle of stings. Bullet ants, which live in central and south America, inflict a sting so painful that it has been compared to being shot.

The bullet ant sting is rated as one of the most painful in the world, according to a four-point scale devised by entomologist Justin Schmidt of the Carl Hayden Bee Research Center in Tucson, Arizona. The Schmidt Sting Pain Index[46] is based on Schmidt's own experience of being voluntarily stung by almost every bee, wasp and ant known to science. Level one pain is mild and ephemeral. Level two is the classic wasp/bee sting experience. Level three is intense, and level four described as 'torture'. Alongside the bullet ant, only two other insects are categorised as level four stingers: the warrior wasp and the tarantula hawk, which is actually a wasp that eats tarantulas. So if you thought a wasp sting was painful, get some perspective.

There are numerous folk remedies for wasp, bee and ant stings. They mostly don't work. Wash them with soapy water to remove any residual venom and put some soothing cream on them.

Bites and stings of all sorts are usually quite harmless and will clear up after a few days, though some people have an allergic reaction. Very occasionally the immune system can go into overdrive and lead to life-threatening anaphylactic shock. If you experience difficulty breathing, dizziness, severe swelling or nausea and vomiting after receiving a bite or sting, seek urgent medical attention. While shouting 'Fly, sore!' at the top of your voice.

Sea urchins and jellyfish

I developed an abiding fear of dangerous sea creatures aged six, during a family holiday on the Italian island of Elba. We were staying in what I considered to be an excellent hotel, largely due to the dessert trolley, but about which my parents had a different opinion.

The seaside was rocky, which was hazardous enough. But it was made doubly dangerous by dark, spiny underwater blobs that carpeted every rock. These turned out to be sea urchins which my dad said had to be avoided at all costs; if you stood on one, the spines stick in your foot and inject deadly poison and you may have to have your leg amputated below the knee.

My dad promptly stood on an urchin, and spent the rest of the holiday removing thick black spines from the ball of his foot. We didn't have any antiseptic – it was the 1970s – so he used cheap Italian plonk, alternately dabbing his spiked foot and taking swigs. His lower leg is still attached to his body, so I think the amputation thing was an exaggeration.

Standing on an urchin really hurts, inflicting what has been described as 'an immediate, incapacitating burning pain'. The advice is to remove the spines as soon as possible and immerse the affected foot in hot water. Or wine.

Some species have venom in their spines which can cause extra pain plus, sometimes, dizziness, nausea, vomiting, breathing difficulties, seizures and, occasionally, cardiac arrest. It goes without saying that if you develop any of these after standing on a sea urchin, go to hospital. But don't expect an antivenom like you might get for a snake bite. There aren't any.

Some urchins also inject an inky substance that stays in the skin long after the spines have been removed, a phenomenon known as tattooing.

Another hazard of swimming is jellyfish stings. Numerous species of jellyfish sting and usually cause no more than pain and a swollen rash or welt. However, some are deadly and, again, if you develop symptoms other than pain and swelling after being stung, seek urgent medical help.

Jellyfish are a hazard all over the world. The worst I am likely to encounter in British waters is the aptly named mauve stinger (*Pelagia noctiluca*), also called the Purple People Eater because of its nasty, though ultimately harmless, sting. We also get the occasional Portuguese man-o'-war (*Physalia physalis*), which can deliver a really nasty and sometimes even fatal sting from its amazingly long tentacles, which can trail up to 20 metres behind it. They get their name because they resemble a jellyfish disguised as an eighteenth-century Portuguese warship, but are not actually jellyfish. They are a floating colony of small jellyfish-like animals called hydrozoa.

There are no records of anyone ever being stung to death by a jellyfish (or similar) in British waters, though never say never. A handful of people elsewhere have been killed by Portuguese man-o'-war stings, and these floating terrors are reportedly becoming more common around Britain as the seas warm up due to climate change. In September 2017, swimming was temporarily banned at Perranporth in Cornwall after a large number of Portuguese men-o'-war washed up on the beach. The UK's Wildlife Trust asks anyone who sees a Portuguese man-o'-war – which, incidentally, are called *caravela-Portuguesa* in Portuguese (caravela were small and highly-manoeuvrable sailing ships developed in the fifteenth century) – to report them to the authorities.

Jellyfish (and similar) stings are specialised cells on the tentacles called nematocysts. These are studded with booby traps: long venomous barbs like microscopic grappling hooks, which are normally coiled up tightly in the nematocyst membrane but if triggered by contact uncoils explosively and shoot outwards, lodging in the skin of whatever triggered them. Some jellyfish constantly shed nematocysts to envelop themselves in a swarm of stingers. These can hang around in the water long after the jelly has drifted off. So the absence of jellies in the sea does not mean you won't get stung.

If you do, don't pee on it. This common remedy, popularised by an episode of *Friends* called 'the one with the jellyfish'[47] where Monica gets stung and Joey offers his services, does not work and can actually exacerbate the pain by causing unexploded barbs to fire. Vinegar also doesn't work. Rinse the site with salt water instead, which is definitely more hygienic and dignified than dousing yourself in pee and has the added virtue of being widely available where jellyfish live.

Worms

My wife's paternal grandmother was, by all accounts, as mad as a bottle of crisps. She came from an Irish family living in the north of England and made her living running a sweet shop in Halifax, West Yorkshire. She was a bit fond of the wine gums, if you get my drift. She also knew her way around the kitchen, both as a cook and a medicine woman.

We've already encountered her way with warts (if you haven't read that section yet, spoiler alert: steal some meat, rub meat on wart, bury meat in the back garden). Now brace yourself for her way with worms. It involved lard. The madcap theory was that if you put some lard in the right place, the worms would pop their heads out, eat lard and die. I know at least three people who were subjected to this bizarre ritual. Where it came from I do not know. At least meat versus warts is a common folk remedy. Lard versus worms, not so much. Coconut oil, yes; maybe lard was the closest thing you could get to that in 1970s Halifax. It was always in the larder, as she was also well-known for her excellent lardy cake. Let's hope she washed her hands in between worming and baking.

The worms that she tried to lard to death were probably pinworms, also called threadworms. These are small parasitic roundworms (nematodes) that live their entire lives in and around the human intestine. They are by far the most common intestinal worms – also called helminths – in Halifax, and indeed the rest of western Europe. Other worms are available, but generate broadly similar symptoms.

Worm infections, also called helminthiases, are generally harmless, though uncomfortable and repulsive. They are also extremely common, especially in children – up to half of children in western countries have them at any one time. Fortunately, they are easily cleared up without spilling a drop of lard.

People usually discover that they are infested by spotting what look like small white pieces of cotton in their faeces. These are dead worms, which are the only good kind. Unfortunately, they are unmistakeable evidence that there are still lots of living ones where the faeces came from. Worms also cause itchiness around the anus. This is caused by – and there is no nice way to say this – female worms crawling out of your arse to lay their eggs. Some people discover that their children have worms by witnessing this spectacle.

The eggs need oxygen to fully mature, which is in short supply on the inside. A single female can incubate 10,000 microscopic eggs, and their centimetre-long bodies become totally crammed with them.

The wiggling of the worms and the presence of their sticky eggs triggers an itch response in what is a very trigger-happy part of the body (see page 77). Once the females have unburdened themselves, they die, and their flaccid corpses end up in poo along with the bodies of the much smaller males that died at home, i.e. in the lower part of the small intestine. But at least they got to have sex first.

What precedes the egg-laying is just as morbidly fascinating. The worms' life cycle starts when a human ingests eggs, perhaps from food that has been touched by somebody with worms who recently itched their itchy arse. This is known as the fecal-oral transmission route. It is how a lot of pathogens go about their business. Worm eggs are very sticky and so can end up being transferred to surfaces and hence onto the hands of a new victim. They are viable for two to three weeks outside a host.

Swallowed eggs pass unscathed through the stomach and into the small intestine, where they hatch after about two weeks. From there the juvenile worms gradually spread throughout the lower reaches of the gut, moulting twice on their way to adulthood, which takes about seven weeks. Once mature they mate and the males drop dead. The females live on for a few more weeks, eating your lunch and gestating their broods. Once ready to lay, they head south.

People with worms often re-infect themselves. I don't need to dwell on the fecal-oral details.

There are many other species of parasitic nematodes, but they all essentially operate in the same manner and cause similar symptoms. And regardless of the specific species, treatment is the same. Oral worming medicines are very effective, and often quite tasty (some are made to resemble sweets or milkshakes so children will swallow them). They contain a helminthicide, usually a compound called mebendazole, which causes the worms' intestines to fall apart so they starve to death. A single dose usually does the trick, but because mebendazole kills the worms but not their eggs a second dose may be needed a couple of weeks later (that will stop the cycle as newly hatched worms are not ready to breed). Treatment does not confer long-term protection, so repeat bouts are common.

As with many human parasites, there are signs that some helminths are developing resistance to mebendazole. But there are plenty of other helminthicides out there so we'll probably be okay.

There are many other types of human-infecting helminth – not just tiny roundworms but also really big ones, plus tapeworms, flatworms (flukes) and spiny-headed worms. Most live in guts but others burrow into the skin or travel around in the bloodstream or lymph system. Fortunately for me, most occur in the tropics and subtropics. Some cause truly horrendous diseases: river blindness, elephantiasis, guinea worm and bilharzia are all caused by worms. People sometimes bring these passengers back from their travels. A few, such as the dwarf tapeworm, are found in temperate regions and are not uncommon. Medical advice is that if you find a large worm in your faeces (and large can mean *large*: the world's most common human helminth, *Ascaris lumbricoides*, is known as 'large roundworm', and for good reason; it can grow up to 35 centimetres) or a section of tapeworm, go see a doctor. Other symptoms of these more serious helminthiases include persistent vomiting and diarrhoea, inexplicable weight loss and an itchy and red worm-shaped rash, especially on the feet. The latter could be caused by soil-dwelling hookworms burrowing into the skin. The roundworms that routinely infect pet dogs and cats can also make do with a human host.

Some people deliberately swallow tapeworm eggs, usually in pill form, in a rather desperate bid to lose weight. It often does not work and just causes the unpleasant side effects of a natural tapeworm infection. When British TV doctor Michael Mosley tried it, he gained weight. He may have lost it again if he had passed the tapeworm in his stool. But after killing his worm with a helminthicide, nothing came out. He assumes it disintegrated and he absorbed it as if it were food.

Which makes lard up the arse sound positively tempting.

When plants attack

During my childhood summer in New Mexico in 1980, I didn't just develop a mortal fear of bugs that wanted to lay their eggs under my skin (mythical) and deadly spiders lurking in woodpiles and toilets (real), but also of another diabolical organism called 'poison ivy'. My American buddies gleefully regaled me with stories of unwary children who became entangled in this awful plant in the woods, and had to be sent home from camp, wherever that was. To a callow ten-year-old from the north of England who liked nothing more than to muck about in the woods, this sounded like something from a scary fairy tale. We had ivy at home, but it wasn't poisonous. What kind of dangerous and terrifying land was this? Then my friends told me about poison oak, and I was ready to pack my bags.

Back home, the worst thing I would encounter in the woods was a nettle. Fortunately, where there were nettles there were bound to be dock leaves, which pretty much proved the existence of God. Nettle stings are not nice, for sure: another of my nephews (not the bee-sting one) once ran headlong into a nettle patch wearing shorts when he was little, and he cried. A lot. But the very definition of nettle is to irritate *a bit*, and nobody ever got sent home from camp because of nettle rash.

There are dozens of plants that answer to the name nettle, many of them as harmless as a blade of grass; some probably evolved to resemble nettles to freeload on the stinging power of the real thing, much like harmless hoverflies that have evolved to look like wasps. This is known as Batesian mimicry after Henry Walter Bates, the biologist who discovered it among butterflies of the Brazilian rainforest, where he travelled with the co-discoverer of natural selection, Alfred Russel Wallace.

The true stinging nettles are a much more select group of plants. Most of them are in the genus *Urtica*, which is derived from *úrere*, the Latin word for 'burn'. The nettle my nephew was stung by is *Urtica dioica*, a perennial flowering plant that originated in Eurasia but is now distributed worldwide.

Nettles sting because they are covered from tip to toe in needle-like hairs called trichomes, which inject a cocktail of irritants into the skin of anyone who as much as brushes against them. This has obviously evolved as a defence mechanism against being eaten, but try telling that to the contestants in the annual World Nettle-Eating Championships, held around the summer solstice at a pub called the Bottle Inn in Marshwood, Dorset. Nettles are traditionally eaten as food but only after boiling or roasting them to neutralise their sting. The championship involves raw, sting-enabled nettles. Contestants have an hour to strip and eat the leaves from as many 2-foot-long stalks as they can. The competition is judged by the length of bare stalks that remain; top competitors regularly eat their way through more than 40 feet of nettles. Then they throw up in the car park, which gets them disqualified.

The way to avoid a nasty rash on the tongue and lips is to munch hard. The trichomes are delicate and easily flattened such that they do not sting. Hence the phrase 'grasp the nettle.'

The irritants in the trichomes include formic acid (which is also found in ant venom, see page 277), the inflammatory compound histamine and the neurotransmitters acetylcholine and serotonin. The latter produces pleasurable feelings in the brain but painful ones in the skin.

Nettle rash is technically called contact urticaria, which is derived from the plant's Latin name and was coined to refer specifically to nettling of the skin. The word 'urticaria' has been extended to any skin rash with red, raised, itchy bumps, known in common parlance as hives. The classic urticaria is a cluster of small white or red raised areas called weals, surrounded by reddened skin called a flare. But hives come in all shapes and sizes. They are usually a sign of an over-zealous immune response to something, including food, medicines, chemicals, allergens (pollen, latex and dust mites are major triggers), heat and infections.

Standard treatment for nettle rash – or hives in general – is anti-itch creams containing antihistamines or hydrocortisone. There is no evidence that dock leaves (another common-or-garden plant name that covers a multitude of species, but the one with nettle-grasping powers is the broadleafed dock *Rumex obtusifolius*) contain any compound that relieves nettle rash, which I daresay throws the existence of God back up into the air. The act of rubbing may help a bit, or may be a source of distraction from the nettle rash.

The skin irritation caused by poison ivy is rather different. The plant – not an actual member of the ivy family, and not even a creeper, but three species of shrubby trees related to pistachios and mangoes – has a toxic cocktail called urushiol in its sap which most people are allergic to. The toxic sap is in the plant's leaves, stems, roots and berries and is easily released. Poison oaks are similarly misnamed. They are not oaks at all but shrubs that are closely related to the poison ivys and contain the same nasty sap.

Skin that comes into contact with urushiol usually becomes red, itchy, painful and blistered, a condition called urushiol-induced contact dermatitis. Blundering into a poison ivy or oak leaf can be enough to release some sap, but urushiol is also remarkably stable and can persist on leaves and twigs for years after leaking out. People who have it on their hands can also contaminate anything they touch, such as doorknobs, worksurfaces and phones, and hence continuously re-inoculate themselves or spread it to other people. This is probably the source of the erroneous belief that the liquid in poison ivy blisters contains (or just is) the poison. It is also why people who have walked through a patch of poison ivy and later remove their shoes can end up with a rash on their hands. The dermatitis – a catch-all name for inflammation of the skin, also called eczema (see page 68) – can last for weeks.

As with nettles, a plant that often grows alongside poison ivy is used as a folk remedy for the rash. But there is no evidence that jewelweed neutralises the sap. Which is yet another blow to the existence of God. And in any case, which benevolent god would create poisonous plants in the first place? On that one, I'm firmly with Wallace and Darwin.

6

Self-Inflicted Wounds

Every year, a group of heroic individuals are honoured for their selfless contribution to human progress. The Darwin Awards are almost always awarded posthumously, which makes sense when you realise what they are for. They 'salute the improvement of the human genome by honouring those who accidentally remove themselves from it in a spectacular manner'. In other words, people who accidentally kill or sterilise themselves (and only themselves) in brainless ways.

Death is hardly a minor illness, so let's leave that there. But there is no doubt that one of the biggest dangers to our health is our own idiocy and carelessness. From falling off ladders to drinking to excess, the finger of blame often points at one person and one person only: ourselves.

Hangovers

An old college mate of mine who I have now lost touch with arrived at university as a somewhat callow youth. He was not an experienced drinker; he had lived a sheltered existence and was not keen on experiencing the morning-after-the-night-before. But he gradually got into the swing of student life and an odd bottle of lager here turned into two or three regular pints there. One night he went on a total bender, aided and abetted by me and the rest of our gang. In the morning he had the full Monty: headache, nausea, vomiting, the shakes and an aversion to bright light and loud noise. He was not a happy bunny, but ever the science geek, one symptom bothered his brain even more than the rest of them tormented his body. 'What I don't understand,' he said, 'is why, even though I drank all night, I'm still so *thirsty*!'

Of all self-inflicted wounds, the hangover is arguably the stupidest. We willingly imbibe a deadly toxin in return for a few hours (at best) of fun followed by a day (or more) of illness. However, as somebody who has inflicted more than his fair share upon himself (irresponsibly; drink sensibly, kids), I also believe there is something magnificently life-affirming about waking up after a long, drunk night of the soul with the feeling that, in the immortal words of Douglas Adams, you have been drunk – as in, how a glass of water feels.

Hangovers are a staple of English literature – no real surprise given the Anglosphere's fondness for the sauce, especially among literary types, and the maxim 'write what you know'. But nobody has ever surpassed Kingsley Amis's description of one in his 1954 novel *Lucky Jim*:[48]

Dixon [Jim] was alive again. Consciousness was upon him before he could get out the way . . . He lay sprawled, too wicked to move, spewed up like a broken spider-crab on the tarry shingle of the morning . . . His mouth has been used as a latrine by some small creature of the night, and then as its mausoleum. During the night, too, he'd somehow been on a cross-country run and then been expertly beaten up by secret police. He felt bad.

That three-letter word is an awfully small description for an awfully big, complex and strangely baffling illness. Medical science recognises forty-seven symptoms of what it officially calls the 'hangover syndrome'. Many have an unknown cause.

But we are getting ahead of ourselves. To become hungover, we have to pass through another phase first: intoxication. The clue is in the name. Somebody who is drunk has definitely consumed a toxin, albeit a beguiling one.

Alcohol – or ethanol, to give it its proper name (there are types of alcohol you definitely don't want to drink, including the deadly toxin methanol, although as we shall see we often do drink it by accident) – is the world's favourite psychoactive drug. It is also the most dangerous, wreaking incomparable damage. In an influential analysis of aggregated drug harms to both individuals and society, the British drug expert David Nutt gave alcohol a score of 72 out of a possible 100.[49] The next worst were heroin (55) and crack cocaine (54). Correct: alcohol is about one-and-a-half times more harmful than crack cocaine.

Despite an often-dysfunctional relationship with ethanol stretching back centuries, we still don't really understand how it weaves its spell. Unlike most psychoactive drugs it does not directly interfere with or enhance any of the brain's signalling pathways, but has an indirect effect on many of them, hence the general and widespread effect of alcohol.

We also know that it has a biphasic effect on the brain. Overall, ethanol is considered a sedative and a hypnotic –

which means it tranquillises us and then sends us to sleep – but in low doses it is a stimulant. This is why a few drinks causes disinhibition, social lubrication and euphoria, but a few more often leads to slurring, swaying, mental confusion, falling over and loss of consciousness. Alcohol also causes temporary amnesia, which can be a bit of a mercy but also a source of morning-after-the-night-before anxiety: what *did* I do last night? This can be exacerbated by the discovery of what a great friend of mine, who used to be able to mix it with the best but has lately given up alcohol completely, called a UDI; an Unidentified Drinking Injury.

And, of course, alcohol causes vomiting. It is a toxin that attracts the attention of an area of the brain called the chemoreceptor trigger zone, which reports to the vomiting centre (see page 193). High levels of blood alcohol also play havoc with the balance system, hence the spinning room phenomenon which is how a night on the tiles can end. Disturbances to this system also wake up the vomiting centre. You might call it a double whuuuurghy.

But still we take the risk, because the potential pain is a price many are prepared to pay for some liquid pleasure. In 1952, the Mississippi state senator Noah S. Sweat (known to his friends as 'Soggy') delivered a famous speech to the state's legislature during a debate on ending prohibition, which was still in force in Mississippi at the time. What became known as the 'whiskey speech' is a brilliant exploration of our double dealings with alcohol. It is too long to reproduce in full, though is worth looking up, but here are edited highlights:

Here is how I feel about whiskey. If when you say whiskey you mean the devil's brew, the poison scourge, the bloody monster . . . then certainly I am against it. But, if when you say whiskey you mean the oil of conversation, the philosophic wine, the ale that is consumed when good fellows get together, that puts a song in their hearts and laughter on their lips, and the warm glow of contentment in their eyes . . . then certainly I am for it. This is my stand. I will not retreat from it. I will not compromise.

The state decided not to repeal prohibition, and stuck to its guns for another fourteen years.

Soggy did not mention hangovers. But no discussion of the poison scourge is complete without discussing them in all their goriness.

Hangovers are indeed a syndrome, meaning a collection of correlated symptoms. In 2012, scientists from the Netherlands approached students on the campus of Utrecht University and asked them to fill in a survey about their most recent hangover.[50] The vast majority agreed even though there was no beer money in it for them. In total the researchers got 1,410 completed surveys. Most of the students did not have to cast their mind too far back, with over half admitting that their most recent hangover was less than a month ago.

The ten most common symptoms they reported were fatigue, thirst, sleepiness, headache, dry mouth, nausea, weakness, reduced alertness, concentration problems and apathy. But there was a long tail of others including sweating, shivering, loss of taste, guilt, regret and confusion.

The main reason why a night on the lash makes us feel ill is – surprise, surprise – the after-effects of imbibing a toxic substance. Many of the top ten symptoms, including headache, nausea, tiredness and apathy, are directly caused by ethanol. Fatigue, meanwhile, is probably down to getting to bed later than normal and then sleeping badly. Like most hypnotic drugs, alcohol knocks us out but does not mimic natural sleep. And when it wears off in the wee small hours (or when we are awoken by the need to wee) we often ping awake and struggle to finish off what was already a poor night's sleep. Dehydration is caused by alcohol's suppression of the antidiuretic hormone vasopressin, which makes you urinate excessively.

Some other symptoms are a bit more mysterious. The delayed onset of hangovers points the finger at the breakdown products of ethanol – especially acetaldehyde, a toxic compound produced by the liver as the first step of breaking down ethanol for disposal.

The vast majority of acetaldehyde is quickly processed to acetate, which is harmless and used for energy by the muscles. But minute amounts of acetaldehyde escape into the bloodstream, where it goes on a bender.

Acetaldehyde is nasty stuff. It reacts irreversibly with proteins and renders them useless; after a booze-up, damaged proteins build up in the liver, muscles, heart, brain and gastrointestinal tract, and contribute to us feeling lousy.

The average liver can process about 7 grams of ethanol an hour, meaning that it takes about twelve hours to chomp through all the ethanol in a bottle of wine. That's twelve hours of continuous exposure to a trickle of poison.

Tobacco smoke also contains acetaldehyde and, anecdotally at least, people who sometimes have a crafty fag with a few drinks say that booze and fags give them a worse hangover than booze alone. Smoking also causes coughs as the lungs try to get rid of all the tar, soot and other nasties, which makes the morning after that bit more of a drag. About half of active smokers have a chronic cough.

Anyway, back to the bottle. Hangovers are also caused in part by 'congeners' – organic compounds other than ethanol produced during fermentation and distillation which contribute deliciously to a drink's district flavour and aroma but also do your head in. They are also called 'fusel oils', from the German word for 'gut rot'. They include methanol.

As a rule of thumb, the darker a drink the more congeners it contains and the greater its hangover potential. And different drinks contain different congeners, which is why mixing drinks is a recipe for rotten guts and more besides.

As for the old adage about 'beer before wine' and 'wine before beer', not only is it impossible to remember which supposedly makes you feel fine/queer, there is no evidence that the order in which we mix drinks makes any difference.

Hangovers anecdotally get worse with age, but recent research suggests the exact opposite. This may be because, like many things in life, practice makes perfect.[51] The livers of frequent drinkers become more efficient at processing ethanol, upping their capacity from 7 grams an hour to 10.

The same research, which used an app to allow drinkers to log their consumption in real time and also their state of body and mind the next day, unsurprisingly confirmed that the main risk factors for a bad hangover are drinking a lot and mixing drinks. It also found that wine produced the worst hangovers.

When it comes to recovery, time is a great healer. There really isn't anything you can do except patiently let the body's natural detoxification and recovery processes run their course. Painkillers, caffeine, water and sleep can help alleviate the discomfort while this twelve- to twenty-four-hour slow torture plays out.

There is no shortage of folk remedies – greasy food, raw eggs, bananas, fresh air, sugary drinks, saunas, vitamins – but there is a shortage of evidence that any of them do any good. Hair of the dog, so-called from the totally useless practice of treating dog bites using a few hairs from the biter, is surprisingly effective in the short term but merely calls a halt on the process of detoxification and so delays and multiplies the inevitable.

Some people find that a punishing workout helps, but again there is scant evidence that it does anything except perhaps atone for the self-loathing that often accompanies a hangover.

The future may bring brighter mornings, however. The aforementioned Professor Nutt has for years been working on alcohol substitutes that give us all the pleasure without most of the pain. And that moment of horrible clarity when we realise we are plastered and that tomorrow is going to be a write-off may soon be an opportunity to take rapid aversive action.

Scientists in Canada recently invented a sobering-up machine that allows people to hyperventilate without passing out.[52] Alcohol is mostly cleared from the bloodstream by the liver, but about 10 per cent is exhaled in breath, and so a period of hyperventilation helps to clear it from the body. Hyperventilation usually causes people to pass out due to respiratory alkalosis, or a dangerous rise in the alkalinity of the blood due to loss of CO_2. The machine returns CO_2 to the blood in just the right quantity to make hyperventilation safe. It is designed for people who have consumed a dangerous amount of alcohol and are at risk of acute alcohol poisoning, but it is a simple device that requires no complex components and could – guys, please? – be turned into a consumer product. 'It's a very basic, low-tech device that could be made anywhere in the world: no electronics, no computers or filters are required,' said its inventor Joseph Fisher, an anaesthesiologist at the Toronto General Hospital Research Institute. 'It's almost inexplicable why we didn't try this decades ago.'

There is, of course, an ethical question mark over a technology that would allow people to drink like fishes then sober up on demand. But I'm prepared to give it the benefit of the doubt. Cheers!

Sports injuries

Exercise is good for you, laziness is not. But there's no gain without pain, and if it ain't hurting, it ain't working. Our bodies have multiple ways of telling us that it's working.

Most exercise-related ailments are simply injuries caused by overdoing it or twisting something; these are called strains and sprains and are damage to muscles and ligaments respectively. The ankle, wrist and knee are prone to sprains as they take a hell of a beating when playing sports. But some are more complicated and mysterious.

Consider the curse of the school cross-country run, the stitch. This intense, stabbing pain can strike without warning and then disappear just as suddenly, usually when you stop running in order to double over in agony. Stitches usually strike on the right side, directly under the ribcage, but can afflict any part of the abdomen and sometimes the shoulder. Being fit is no defence; even though they were once dismissed as an affliction of the 'constitutionally inferior', elite runners also get stitches from time to time.[53] What they are and why they happen is a total head-scratcher.

If the name evokes the sense of being stabbed with a needle, that is no coincidence. It is derived from the Old English word *stiċe*, which meant 'to puncture or prick', and which also gave rise to the word 'stick' (as in a pointy bit of wood) and 'stitch', in the sewing sense.

Stitches are very common; around 70 per cent of people who regularly go running report getting at least one a year, and in any given race about one in five runners gets one. Swimming, horse riding and aerobics are also common causes of what is properly called exercise-related transient abdominal pain (ETAP).

As for explanations, the medical name really says it all. A stitch is abdominal pain that is exercise-related. Beyond that, who knows? There are numerous hypotheses for the underlying cause, but no consensus. The fact that it is usually triggered by forms of exercise requiring repetitive motion of the torso suggest that it may simply be muscle cramp – of which more later. Or maybe it is overstretching of the ligaments attaching the abdominal organs to the diaphragm. Or maybe irritation of the membrane wrapped around the abdominal organs. Or maybe a lack of blood in the diaphragm, or too much blood in the liver or spleen. Or maybe exercising on a full stomach. You get the picture.

As pain goes, stitches are not trivial. On a scale from one to ten, most people rate the intensity as about five. Research on recreational runners suggests that getting a stitch usually causes them to slow down or even stop. But constitutionally superior runners just grit their teeth and run through the pain, which usually goes away of its own accord after a couple of minutes.

One thing exercise physiologists agree on is that exercise-related transient abdominal pain is totally harmless and does not indicate an underlying health problem or lack of fitness. If stitches are getting in the way of your exercise regime, consider switching to cycling, which is the form of endurance exercise least likely to bring one on. Or, according to the tongue-in-cheek advice of Australian sports physiologist Paul McCrory, take up chess or darts or simply 'grow old, as stitches are less common with ageing'.[54]

If stitches really are a form of muscle cramp, then they are just another manifestation of a common and sometimes agonising exercise-related ailment. However, that does not fully solve the mystery of their origin.

The cause of exercise-associated muscle cramps is also not entirely clear. Fatigue and dehydration are clearly factors, hence the common sight of footballers 'going down with cramp' near the end of extra time in the cup final – though maybe they are just trying to avoid having to step up to the spot in a penalty shootout. But exactly why fatigue and/or dehydration cause muscles to cramp remains an unresolved question.

Cramp is simply a muscle contracting involuntarily and very hard, and staying that way for a while. It can be horribly painful, last for hours, and render an entire limb useless.

One explanation is that dehydration caused by sweating leads to an imbalance of electrolytes, which are inorganic compounds such as sodium and chlorine dissolved in the blood. This makes some sort of sense: muscle contraction is triggered by an influx of sodium ions into the muscle cell, followed by a release of stored calcium ions. But how a dearth of sodium or calcium can lead to involuntary contraction has not been adequately explained.

Another hypothesis is that fatigue somehow causes the nerve signals that normally trigger voluntary muscle contraction to go haywire. Again the exact mechanism has not been elucidated, but this is now considered the most plausible hypothesis.

The best way to relieve cramp is to stop exercising – which is pretty much non-negotiable anyway – and try to un-cramp the cramped muscle by stretching it. That is what footballers are doing when they raise a cramp-afflicted team-mate's leg and push down on their foot. Massage can help too.

Cramp is painful but not dangerous, unless it strikes while swimming. Worldwide, there are 1.2 million deaths by drowning each year and cramp is probably a factor in many of them, though exact figures are impossible to obtain for obvious reasons. However, the idea that cramp is caused by getting into the water too soon after eating, when 'all the blood has gone to your stomach', is a myth. Lack of blood does not cause cramp and in any case blood does not 'go to your stomach'. Swimming on a full stomach is no more risky than swimming on an empty one, unless the meal was boozy. Alcohol can cause cramp, so don't drink and dive.

Cramps usually clear up by themselves but often leave a lingering legacy of muscle soreness, which is yet another painful hazard of exercise.

There are three kinds of muscle soreness. The first is acute, which is essentially fatigue: it hurts briefly during and after exercise but soon ebbs away. Then there's the 'pulled muscle' or muscle strain which is caused by damage to the muscle tissue and may take weeks to heal; and finally delayed-onset muscle soreness, or DOMS, which is a bit of both.

DOMS is the pain and stiffness that usually start to bother you a day or two after a vigorous workout and can render you almost immobile for a couple of days. The usual explanation is a build-up of lactic acid. This does happen during exercise but is definitively not the source of your pain. DOMS is actually the result of minor tears and ruptures of overworked muscle fibres, which can lead to temporary inflammation. But, again, no pain, no gain. The repair processes that fix the damage make the muscle a little bit stronger and bigger, so that an identical workout will be slightly easier next time and render you slightly less stiff afterwards. And you will have bigger, stronger muscles.

The dreaded dead leg is another form of muscular injury common on contact sports. It is inflicted by a sharp blow to the frontal thigh muscle by an object such as a knee or football boot which crushes the muscle against the femur and damages it. The leg can go numb and immobile, hence 'dead'. It isn't: rest, ice, compression and elevation will miraculously bring it back to life. In a week or so.

Shin splints are another painful consequence of exercise, and seem especially cruel as they usually afflict unfit people who have recently vacated the couch and taken up running. They cause pain and tenderness along the edges of the shin bones, especially while pounding the pavement. The underlying problem is inflammation from repeatedly striking a hard surface. The solution is to take painkillers, apply ice and take a break from the exercise that caused them. Once the pain has gone (and assuming the motivation is still there), gradually go back to running, preferably on a soft surface.

Contact sports such as rugby and martial arts present yet another hazard: having the wind knocked out of you. A blow to the upper abdomen or back, such as when a massive prop forward clatters into you or a black belt judoka flings you to the ground like a rag doll, can cause temporary shutdown of a bunch of nerves in the abdomen commonly called the solar plexus but technically called the celiac plexus. This can temporarily paralyse the diaphragm, making it extremely difficult to breathe. Being winded is a frightening and unpleasant experience, especially when you're already short of breath through exertion, but will go away in a few minutes.

Another blow that will knock the stuffing out of you (if you are a man) is a kick or knee in the testicles. 'It is common knowledge that any blow to the scrotum produces severe pain,' wrote a doctor called Anita Bell in a 1961 article called 'Some observations on the role of the scrotal sac and testicles'.[55] The testicles are rich in nerve endings and, aside from the thick wrinkly skin of the scrotum, are unprotected. The pain of a blow to the crown jewels can radiate into the abdomen, from whence the testicles descended and to which they are still attached, and can be bad enough to induce vomiting. But unless some lasting damage has been done – which it goes without saying needs urgent medical attention – the pain fades after an hour or so. Professional sportsmen often wear protection, or at least put their hands over their nether regions when facing a free kick. Cricket is a major threat; you do not want to take a fast-moving cricket ball in the balls, and not just because that can get you out LBW. Batsmen and wicket keepers routinely wear very solid groin guards. Women cricketers often wear them too; they call them 'manhole covers'.

You may conclude that all this agony simply isn't worth the aggro and opt for laziness. But the long-term risks of not exercising are much greater than any short-term discomfort. The mantra bears repeating: no pain, no gain.

Sunstroke and sunburn

I've had radiation sickness twice, and would not recommend it. The first time was in France and I was as sick as a dog for days. The second time was in Greece; that time I caught it early and cured myself with a whacking dose of dihydrogen monoxide. The source of the radiation in both cases was a gigantic ball of plasma heated to about 5,500°C by nuclear fusion reactions in its core.

Okay, I'm exaggerating. I had common-or-garden sunstroke, or heat exhaustion as it is properly known. The cause was thermal radiation – also called heat – and the source was the sun. But it was still horrible. And I did successfully use dihydrogen monoxide (chemical formula H_2O) to cure it.

Heat exhaustion is no great mystery. It is caused by overheating. When the weather is very hot, or our bodies generate way too much heat through extreme exertion, the normal thermoregulatory mechanisms that keep us cool are overwhelmed. Core body temperature soars to dangerous levels of 40°C or more, and things start to break down. The symptoms – aside from feeling very hot – are dizziness, confusion, extreme thirst, nausea and vomiting, muscle cramps, fatigue, heavy sweating and pale clammy skin.

These are all warning signs to cool it, pronto. If heat exhaustion goes on for more than thirty minutes it can progress to heatstroke, which is a medical emergency. Get out of the sun, drink plenty of cold water, apply ice packs and, if possible, take a long cold shower. When I got it in Greece I stood, shivering, under a cold trickle for about half an hour (Greece may be the cradle of western civilisation, but the cradle of quality plumbing it ain't). Then I felt fine and went out for a couple of ouzos.

Incidentally, I learned the cold shower cure from a vet* who told me how he once diagnosed a poorly bull with heat stroke and cured him with a hose pipe.

Actual heatstroke can be fatal, as prolonged excess heat damages vital organs. One warning sign is, paradoxically, a cessation of sweating despite feeling very hot. Shortness of breath, mental confusion and seizures too. Get help.

When I got sunstroke in France, aged about ten, my dad told me it was caused by gamma rays from the sun frazzling my brain, which at least seemed quite cool as I shivered in bed waiting for the next attack of vomiting. Cool, but rubbish. This is a popular misconception and is the main reason why people wear hats in the sun. But think about it: if gamma rays can penetrate a mop of hair and a skull, a hat isn't going to stop them. And in any case sunlight does not contain gamma rays.

Nonetheless, a hat can help prevent heat exhaustion by taking the brunt of the heat. As can anything that keeps us cool. Sunscreen is a good idea as it soaks up some of the thermal energy beating down from the rather unremarkable star at the centre of our solar system. Staying out of the midday star in the first place is also a clever idea. But try telling that to an Englishman on his summer holidays. Mad dogs and all that.

Heat exhaustion is one of several illnesses caused by excessive heat, collectively known as (surprise!) heat illnesses. One is heat syncope, or fainting, as perfected by soldiers Trooping the Colour while wearing fur hats in a heatwave; not all hats are created equal when it comes to staying cool. Heat cramps can result from loss of salt through excessive sweating.

---

* Via the medium of a book called *All Creatures Great and Small*. The vet was James Wight, better known by his pen name James Herriot.

Another is prickly heat, also called heat rash or sweat rash, which I've never had but my younger son says is agony. It happens when sweat glands become clogged and sweat gets trapped in them. With nowhere else to go, the sweat is forced to burst out into the underlying skin. It is characterised by the sudden appearance of a prickly red rash and/or blisters on the skin. At its worst it can cause what is known as 'wild-fire', with painful lesions spreading like, well, wildfire all over the body. As sweating is a key element of thermoregulation, prickly heat can make heat exhaustion more likely.

It can be calmed down with damp cloths, ice packs and soothing lotions, but the best solution is to avoid it in the first place. Stay cool. Drink dihydrogen monoxide. And exfoliate.

And, of course, wear sunscreen. Another form of radiation damage that I have carelessly and stupidly endured many times is sunburn. In this case, the damage is done by ultraviolet B, or UVB, an invisible form of high(ish)-energy electromagnetic radiation that streams out of the sun and dumps energy onto whatever is in its way, including bare skin. Even though sunshine is hot, sunburn is not a thermal burn like you might get from touching a hot coal (see page 113). It is more like a radiation burn that you might get from, say, Chernobyl. The UVB penetrates the upper layer of skin and damages the DNA inside skin cells. Sunburn is the body's emergency response to this potentially dangerous genetic damage.

The frontline defence is inflammation, which causes the redness and pain. It is cleverly designed to lower the skin's tolerance to heat, making further sun exposure painful and motivating us to take shelter. Unburned skin starts to hurt at about 43°C but burned skin will scream out at 30°C.

DNA repair processes also kick in, but the damage can sometimes be irreparable. Cells with irredeemably damaged DNA execute a suicide programme called apoptosis, which prevents them from becoming cancerous. Dying cells contribute to the pain and redness, and once these acute effects have passed entire sheets of dead skin may slough off. Sunburn can take several days to subside.

If exposure to UVB is very prolonged or UVB levels are very high, the damage can penetrate into deeper layers of the skin and lead to blistering, as inflammation and cell suicide run amok.

The least responsive of the body's defence reactions is production of brown and black pigments called melanins, which are designed to absorb punishing doses of UVB without falling apart and so provide a shield for DNA. It can take fair skin a week or more of prolonged UVB exposure to build up noticeable levels of melanin, also known as a suntan.

Tanned skin feels and looks nice, so people are often prepared to endure a day or two of mild sunburn to expedite the tanning process. Bad idea. Every dose of sunburn increases the probability of a cell accumulating just the right sort of DNA damage to turn it cancerous without tripping its suicide programme. Hence the strong correlation between getting burned and getting skin cancer, which is frighteningly lethal. In a bid to become brown, you may end up brown bread instead.

Sunlight also contains the slightly-lower-energy UVA, which burns a bit but is mainly thought to contribute to the skin-ageing effect of prolonged sun exposure. It can also inflict DNA damage and stimulate melanin production. About 95 per cent of the UV in sunlight is UVA, so even though it is weaker it can still pack a punch.

Depending on how fair-skinned we are, sunburn can develop after as little as ten minutes of exposure, but usually takes an hour or so. Naturally dark skin is much more resistant but will burn eventually. Once burned, you are in for an uncomfortable ride. The inflammation and soreness are going to get worse for up to forty-eight hours even without further exposure, then gradually fade. Itchy peeling often follows.

There is no cure for sunburn, though dermatologists recommend frequent cold baths or showers and moisturiser. The sap of *Aloe vera* – a succulent plant native to the Arabian peninsula – is often applied to sunburn. It has soothing cooling properties but there is absolutely no evidence that it does anything to speed up recovery.[56] It also doesn't block UV. Don't wear aloe vera as sunscreen.

Sunburn is easily avoided with a bit of effort. Clothes and hats cut out UV, which is strongest and most dangerous when the sun is high in the sky. Sunscreen is also highly effective, because it contains compounds not dissimilar to melanin that absorb UVB before it can smash up DNA. Some sunscreens are more protective than others. In case you have been living under a rock since 1974 when the system was invented, the protectiveness of a sunscreen is measured by its SPF rating, or 'sun protection factor'. This is an index of how much of the UV will be filtered out, assuming the sunscreen is applied properly. SPF20, for example, allows one-twentieth of the UVB through. This system also allows sunbathers to calibrate their exposure to the sun. Somebody who typically burns after fifteen unprotected minutes should be able to stay unfrazzled for five hours. But DNA damage still occurs before sunburn hits, so be sensible. And take any claims of waterproofiness with a pinch of sunshine: several studies have shown those claims to be unreliable.

So if sunburn and the risk of deadly cancer is not your idea of a sunny day out, follow the advice of the hit novelty song from 1999 and 'wear sunscreen.'* What that song failed

---

* The song is called 'Everybody's Free (to Wear Sunscreen)', by Baz Luhrmann. It is often said to have been inspired by a speech the author Kurt Vonnegut gave at the Massachusetts Institute of Technology, but the words are actually an essay called 'Advice, Like Youth, Probably Just Wasted on the Young' written by *Chicago Tribune* columnist Mary Schmich. That essay also contains the sage advice, 'Be kind to your knees – you'll miss them when they're gone.'

to mention is that to attain the advertised SPF, the sunscreen must be applied evenly at a concentration of 2 milligrams per square centimetre of skin. Wear sunscreen, but don't forget to bring a ruler and graduated pipette.

Dehydration

Everybody knows you should drink eight glasses of water a day. What nobody knows is where that advice originated from, how big the glass is supposed to be, or how it became such a well-known medical fact. It may be the world's most successful marketing message, except that no one can recall which brand of mineral water started the campaign. In 2002, physiologist Heinz Valtin of Dartmouth Medical School in New Hampshire tried to track down the wellspring of the eight-glasses-a-day meme but failed to find it.[57]

If anything, the number is too low. The US Institute of Medicine recommends 2.7 litres of water a day for women and 3.7 litres for men, to top up what is lost through urine, sweat and breath. That is eight pretty big glasses – about six and a half pints for a man.

However, the Institute also points out that all drinks count. Tea, coffee, juice, sodas and even some alcoholic drinks all contribute. Contrary to common belief, caffeinated drinks do not cause us to pee out more fluid than we take in. Caffeine is a moderate diuretic but not to the extent that it is dehydrating. Ditto alcohol, as long as we stick to beer and other weak drinks. Indeed, weak beer – also called 'small beer', about 1 per cent alcohol – was for centuries the everyday drink of choice for the multitudes, including children, as it was safer than bacteria-laced water. In Sweden, which has some of the most restrictive alcohol laws in the western world, it still is. Even though drinks that are more than 3.5 per cent alcohol by volume are only available in the government-owned liquor chain called Systembolaget, beer up to 2.25 per cent alcohol is treated as a soft drink, sold in grocery stores with no age restrictions, and often served in company canteens at lunch time. Skål!

The water in food also contributes. Some 20 to 30 per cent of an average person's fluid intake is from food. Even some very dry foods are quite watery. A dry cracker is about 10 per cent water. But still, they are not a particularly good way to stay hydrated.

A lot of people are excessively afraid of becoming dehydrated, but it is very easy not to. According to the Food and Nutrition Board of the US National Academies of Science, Engineering and Medicine, most healthy people easily meet their daily water needs by letting thirst be their guide. Even intense exercise will rarely lead to dehydration unless it is hot and there is no access to water. In other words, there really is no need to push the fluids, unless you are a fan of frequent urination.

In fact, fluid-pushers are often found to have too little sodium in their blood, a state called mild hyponatremia. This is not a major issue, but has been associated with mild cognitive impairment.

Dehydration is also not pleasant – it causes dizziness (see page 239), headaches, fatigue, and (shock horror) thirst. But it is as easily cured as it is avoided, by letting your body be your guide. When the thirst is quenched, you will be cured. There's really no need to sweat about it.

Paper cuts

Viz comic once ran a spoof story headlined 'Scientists Discover Worst Thing'. It reported how a team at the University of Budapest had tested all sorts of dreadful things, including pulling out teeth and toenails, but found that nothing was worse than a paper cut on a certain part of a gentleman's anatomy.

The fact that paper can cut skin at all, and with such painful results, is a bit incongruous. But as anyone who has sliced a finger while photocopying or opening an envelope knows, the edge of a sheet of paper can be surprisingly dangerous. The disproportionate pain can be explained by the fact that the cuts are usually (phew) on fingertips, which have high concentrations of pain receptors. They also rarely bleed – paper may be sharp and rigid, but not to the extent that it can slice through blood vessels – and bleeding plugs a wound and protects it from further trauma. Paper cuts also look clean but the edge is more like a saw than a razor blade and will often deposit wood fibres into the wound.

There are no reports in the medical literature of a paper cut to that part of the anatomy. But according to dermatologist Dr Hayley Goldbach of the University of California, quoted in a BBC *Focus* article about paper cuts, 'It would probably also hurt a lot if you got a paper cut in your genitals.' *Viz*, we salute you.

Razor burn

In his brilliant book *Sum: Forty Tales from the Afterlives*, neuroscientist David Eagleman imagines forty different fates that might await us once we are dead. In one, God is the size of a bacterium and is unaware of human existence. In another, the dead play parts in living people's dreams. In yet another we relive our lives but in a different order: every moment we spent on each type of experience is bunched together. So we spend 200 days in the shower, fifteen months looking for things we have lost, eighteen days staring into the refrigerator, six months watching TV commercials, and so on.

One thing Eagleman omitted to add up was shaving. I reckon that would occupy about two months, after which the razor burn would be terrible. Shaving is a tedious but also quite risky activity. It involves dragging a razor-sharp piece of metal across the delicate and weirdly contoured skin of whatever part of the body we are attempting to depilate, which means scything through shafts of the hair as close to the skin as possible (total uprooting of hair by tweezers, etc. is called epilation). The risk of nicks and cuts is substantial, as is the risk of leaving the house with bloody scraps of toilet paper still stuck to the face. And even if the shave is clean in that respect, there's still the risk of a rash or razor burn.

The cause of such a rash is no mystery: damage to the surface of the skin by scraping a razor across it, which is a form of irritant contact dermatitis (see page 68). Blunt razors, pressing too hard and un-lubricated skin increase the burn. Good preparation, careful and gentle shaving with the grain of the hair, warm water and not reshaving an already shaved area all reduce the risk. But once the damage is done, it's done.

A post-shave moisturiser will help soothe the dermatitis but there's not a lot you can do except give it time to heal. And then risk doing it all over again to remove the stubble that grew in the meantime.

Shaving can also lead to pseudofolliculitis barbae, or ingrowing hairs (see page 63), especially in people with thick and tightly coiled body hair. The sliced-through hair can head off in the wrong direction and burrow back into the follicle, causing an inflamed pimple called a razor bump. The only sure-fire solution is to stop shaving. Thus freeing up time for something more fun to repeat again on the other side.

Household injuries

Safe as houses? Forget it. According to the British charity Royal Society for the Prevention of Accidents, home is where the danger is. Every year 2.7 million British people turn up at A&E after an accident at home; 6,000 people a year die from household accidents. Injuries sustained at home are far more common than occupational ones or even road accidents. When a hospital in England decided to compile some stats, it found that around 40 per cent of people who came into A&E with an injury had sustained it at home, compared with 15 per cent who had been hurt on the road and just 8 per cent at work.[58]

The most common household accident is falling. People fall off ladders, out of windows and lofts, trip on carpets and wires and slip on wet floors. Trampolines are especially common things to fall off, especially if adults and children are on them at the same time, as heavier bouncers can catapult lighter ones over the edge.

DIY takes a heavy toll. About 200,000 British people end up in A&E each year after a botched home improvement job or ill-fated gardening project, roughly four out of five of them men. The Easter weekend is a notorious time for such accidents: as the murk of winter lifts, an atavistic desire to clean and fix things courses through our veins and blokes up and down the land decide it is time to get their tools out, often after lunch in the pub. Don't drink and DIY.

The most common DIY accident is falling off a ladder; about 60 per cent of such falls result in a broken bone. Wallpapering and tiling are very hazardous, as trying to do something as challenging as hanging wallpaper or grouting while not falling off a wobbly stepladder is even harder than walking and chewing gum. Tools are dangerous; they are often designed for cutting through materials much tougher than human flesh, and hand trauma from saws, hammers, drills, chisels and power tools are the second most common injuries after falls. Some people injure themselves with a tool they are holding as they fall off a ladder.

Eye injuries are also common in people using power tools without putting on goggles first. But don't improvise. Swimming goggles can be dangerous if you pull them off your face to demist them and accidentally let go.[59]

Gardens are also not for the faint hearted.[60] One of the fictitious heavy metal band Spinal Tap's ill-fated drummers died in a bizarre gardening accident, but in reality such accidents are no joke. About 90,000 people a year in Britain require hospital treatment after injuring themselves while doing the garden. Lawnmowers and electric hedge trimmers are the number one hazard, followed by being hit on the head by falling objects such as sawn-off tree branches and flower pots. Secateurs, spades, hoes, shears and garden forks are an obvious hazard, though unfortunately there are no official statistics on how many people get smacked in the face after standing on the wrong end of a garden fork. About 2,000 people end up in hospital as a result of tangling with a hosepipe.

The kitchen is another death trap, unsurprisingly. Everywhere you turn there are blades, fire, hot things, scalding liquid, glass and electrical appliances, not to mention a collection of noxious substances under the sink. The floor can be wet and people often cook while drunk. About half of household injuries are cooking-related and a further 6 per cent are poisonings when people – usually children – drink bleach, eat rat pellets or inhale glue.

One notorious cooking injury is avocado hand, caused by a cack-handed attempt to remove the stone from an avocado using the tip of a sharp knife. In 2017, the British Association of Plastic, Reconstructive, and Aesthetic Surgeons (not to be confused with the British Association of Aesthetic Plastic Surgeons, also known by the acronym BAAPS, which is appropriate given that they do a lot of boob jobs) highlighted the danger of pointy blades slipping on greasy avocado stones and plunging into the fleshy part of the hand. The association called for avocados to carry a warning label and instructions on how to safely remove the stone. 'There is minimal understanding of how to handle them,' honorary secretary Simon Eccles told *The Times* newspaper.

There is another common category of household injury that involves foreign objects becoming lodged in locations they were not designed to fit into. This often involves small toys and children's nostrils or earholes but there are adult versions too. I need not elaborate.

For the record, the recommended way to remove an avocado stone is to chop into it with the blade of a big, sharp knife and twist. What could possibly go wrong?

Hypochondria

Doctor: 'I think you've got hypochondria.'
Patient: 'Oh no, not that as well!'

People who constantly fret that they are poorly are easy to joke about, but full-blown hypochondria is no laughing matter. Obsessive preoccupation with the possibility of having one or more serious diseases is both exhausting and debilitating.

But to some extent we are all hypochondriacs. The line between normal, healthy concern about our health and the all-consuming anxiety disorder known as hypochondriasis is a blurry one. Who hasn't read or heard about a health condition and thought, that's me! During the writing of this book, I experienced mild anxiety about all manner of minor health conditions, occasionally with good reason. As the comedian Spike Milligan wanted to have etched on his gravestone, 'I told you I was ill!'*

I have certainly found that writing about, say, headaches or nausea or itching or coughing is a pretty reliable trigger of those exact same symptoms. This takes us into the somewhat murky scientific territory of psychosomatic disease, which is basically thinking yourself ill. Many diseases have a psychological component but whether or not it is possible for a physical disease to be all in your head remains controversial.

However, being slightly worried about one's health is

---

* The church was apparently unhappy with this request so Milligan's family came up with a delightfully Milliganesque solution, engraving the stone with the epithet *'Dúirt mé leat go raibh mé breoite'*. This is Gaelic for 'I told you I was ill.'

actually rational and healthy, as catching things early is better than letting them linger. If you think you are ill, my advice is to get it checked out. But if you find yourself ruminating about the possibility of being ill, endlessly checking for signs of illness, and seeking reassurance that you are not ill, it might be time to make a self-diagnosis. Of hypochondria. Which leads me to another slightly meta joke. 'Doctor, doctor, I think I'm a hypochondriac.'

In popular culture, men are more likely than women to grumble about their health, and to exaggerate their symptoms if they are actually ill, such as insisting they have flu when all that is wrong is a cold. This 'man flu' is a global phenomenon and is not entirely implausible. Women generally have stronger immune systems than men by virtue of having two mighty X-chromosomes rather than one X and one weak and snivelling Y (yes, men are genetically stunted). One of the two X-chromosomes in a female cell is switched off, a process called X-inactivation. But for reasons unknown a few genes remain active, including some that are involved in the immune response – notably a gene called TLR7, which makes a protein that detects viruses. Women therefore have a stronger anti-viral immune response than men, and men are known to get sicker and die more often from some viral diseases, including influenza and Covid-19. We told you we were ill . . .

It is certainly possible to escalate concerns about genuine symptoms by reading about them. When done on the internet this is known as cyberchondria. In old-fashioned book form I guess we should call it bibliochondria. If I have triggered it in you too, I apologise. But hey, I have also done you a favour. The next time you get caught in inevitable small talk about minor ailments, you'll be the smartest person in the room, or knowledgeable enough to bore everyone into changing the subject. And you'll hopefully be healthier. As the old saying goes, what doesn't kill you only makes you stronger. Stay alive.

Epilogue

It took me the best part of a year to write this book and what a year it has been! I can confirm that I have not been a well man. I haven't gone down with anything that sent me crawling under the duvet, but my *Mustn't Grumble* diary (which I have now retired, hurt) shows that not a single day went by without there being something small to sweat about. A blocked nose here and a pimple there, a few injuries from cooking and DIY, a hangover and an Unidentified Drinking Injury (see page 296) or two. A lot of excess flatus, a spot of sunburn and multiple banged funny bones (now I've finished writing I might find time to remove that cursed bracket). My tinnitus has got worse and I have developed a whole new repertoire of earworms. And of course there's been the cyberchondria.

But in November 2020 I did have a proper health scare. I suddenly lost my sense of taste. I made a tuna sandwich for my lunch and it tasted of cardboard. Uh oh, I thought: my son had recently recovered from a bout of Covid-19 he caught at university and the first thing he noticed was a lost sense of taste.

I went to the kitchen and tried some other foods. An orange tasted like water. Cheese was like chalk. Chilli sauce had a kick but no flavour. I will admit that I was scared. I could get seriously ill here, I thought. Or even die. And even if I survived what I had now convinced myself was an open-and-shut case of Covid-19, I could be in for the long haul. I went and got a test; sixty anxious (and tasteless) hours later it came back negative. *Memento mori*.

I celebrated with a toasted cheese sandwich and it tasted magnificent.

The experience took me back to the day I sat in a bustling coffee shop in central London, in the Before Times when that felt like the most ordinary thing in the world to do, talking to my agent Toby about an idea for a book on minor ailments. At the time it was increasingly clear that there was something brewing on the distant horizon that could develop into a global health catastrophe. It did not feel like an auspicious moment to be pitching a book about sniffles and warts. Toby thought so too.

Why would anyone at this moment in history, he asked, pointedly, want to read about minor ailments? Because by the time it is done, I said, winging it, we'll be back to sweating the small stuff.

Now, in January 2021, as I put the finishing touches to the first draft, that feels luckily prescient. The first mass vaccination programmes for Covid-19 are being rolled out and it looks very much like the coronavirus that has caused so much suffering and disruption is on its way to becoming just another annoying virus among many. I obviously don't know where we will be when this book is published – the events of 2020 have shown the folly of making predictions, and there is still a long way to go – but I believe that by the time it comes out, we will be looking back at a pandemic receding in the rear-view mirror rather than one looming ahead of us.

I will make one prediction, however: the experience of living through a pandemic will have changed all of us for good – in both senses of the word. Never again will a cough, mild fever or slight change in taste or smell seem like something to not grumble about. Our safe space has been invaded by a deadly pathogen that has dragged us back to a world where somebody with a sniffle, cough or fever can be gravely ill or even dead in a week.

As a result, never again will we take for granted that wondrous state of affairs where the vast majority of us live for seventy-five or eighty-five years with little more serious than a bout of the flu or a broken bone to contend with. As I said at the start, I regard these as the price we all pay for the staggeringly unlikely privilege of being alive at all, and mostly well enough to enjoy it.

I'm fifty-one and will be knocking on the door of fifty-two by the time this book comes out. I reckon I have at least thirty years left on the clock, but however many I get I intend to enjoy them. *Memento mori*. Or, if I may offer up a Latin neologism of my own, *neque murmuraveritis*.[*]

---

[*] For those whose Latin is rusty, or (like me) went to an ordinary school, this translates as 'must not grumble'.

Acknowledgements

I'm not one for ancestor worship, but this book would not have been possible without countless generations of humans, proto-humans, mammals, synapsids, tetrapods, bony fishes, early chordates and unicellular animals all the way back to LUCA, the Last Universal Common Ancestor. The human body and all of its ills are a product of 3.5 billion years of evolution. I am indebted to every one of those life forms that survived and reproduced. Especially a pair of hairless anthropoid apes otherwise known as my parents.

Thanks, too, to all of the viruses, bacteria, archaea, fungi, parasites, insects, bugs and arachnids that have evolved to make a living sponging off humans. Without you, our travails would be much less interesting.

Thanks also to my family and friends for supplying me with so much material – there was more than I could use and if your story didn't make it, apologies. Be slightly ill in a more interesting way next time!

I'm gutted that the signature illness of my best friend Gareth did not make it in, cut from the manuscript on the grounds that London's Disease – a rather unpleasant combination of hangover, malnutrition and sleep deprivation caused by a weekend bender – is not a real disease. I will be lobbying the medical authorities to have it officially recognised.

I'm also extremely grateful to my agent Toby Mundy for believing in this project, and to Lindsey Evans, Kate Miles and Lindsay Davies at Headline Home for helping me bring it to fruition.

And last but not least to my ever-brilliant colleagues and friends at *New Scientist,* both present and past, for constantly reminding me how wonderful and fascinating science is, and for writing excellent books that inspired me to try to do the same.

Endnotes

1 https://ichd-3.org/other-primary-headache-disorders/
4-3-primary-headache-associated-with-sexual-activity/

2 https://ichd-3.org/

3 Stovner, L. J.; Hagen, K.; Jensen, R. et al., 'The Global Burden of Headache: A Documentation of Headache Prevalence and Disability Worldwide', *Cephalagia*, 27(3), pp. 193–210 (2007). DOI: 10.1111/j.1468-2982.2007.01288.x

4 Rizzoli, P.; Mullally, W. J., 'Headache', *The American Journal of Medicine*, 131(1), pp. 17–24 (2018). DOI: 10.1016/j.amjmed.2017.09.005

5 Friedman, A. P., 'The Headache in History, Literature, and Legend', *Bulletin of the New York Academy of Medicine*, 48(4), pp. 661–81 (1972). PMCID: PMC1806702

6 Schwartz, B. S.; Stewart W. F.; Simon, D. et al., 'Epidemiology of Tension-Type Headache', *JAMA*, 279(5) pp. 381–3 (1998). DOI: 10.1001/jama.279.5.381

7 https://www.who.int/news-room/q-a-detail/how-common-are-headaches

8 Ibid.

9 Seeger, S., 'Tension-Type Headache', in Abd-Elsayed, A. (ed.), *Pain: A Review Guide*, Springer, Cham (2019). DOI: 10.1007/978-3-319-99124-5_123

10 Antonelli, M.; Donelli, D.; Valussi, M., 'Efficacy, Safety and Tolerability of Tiger Balm® Ointments: A Systematic Review and a Meta-Analysis of Prevalence', *Journal of Pharmacy & Pharmacognosy Research*, 8(1), pp. 1–17 (2020). http://jppres.com/jppres/pdf/vol8/jppres19.716_8.1.1.pdf

11 Ibid.

12 https://www.nidcr.nih.gov/research/data-statistics/dental-caries/adults

13 Al Aboud, A. M.; Nigam, P.K., 'Wart', *StatPearls*, StatPearls Publishing (2017)

14 https://www.sciencedirect.com/topics/medicine-and-dentistry/sebaceous-gland

15 Robles-Tenorio, A.; Tarango-Martinez, V.M.; Sierra-Silva, G. 'Aquagenic urticaria: Water, friend, or foe?', Clinical Case Reports, 8(11). pp. 2121–2124 (2020). DOI: 10.1002/ccr3.2880

16 Wang, F.; Kim, B. S., 'Itch: A Paradigm of Neuroimmune Crosstalk', Immunity, 52(5), pp. 753–66 (2020). DOI: 10.1016/j.immuni.2020.04.008

17 Mailler, E. A.; Adams, B. B., 'The Wear and Tear of 26.2: Dermatological Injuries Reported on Marathon Day', British Journal of Sports Medicine, 38(4), pp. 498–501 (2004). DOI: 10.1136/bjsm.2004.011874

18 Jurk, K.; Walter, U., 'New Insights into Platelet Signalling Pathways by Functional and Proteomic Approaches', Hamostaseologie, 39(02), pp. 140–51 (2019). DOI: 10.1055/s-0038-1675356

19 Drosou, A.; Falabella, A.; Kirsner, R. S., 'Antiseptics on Wounds: An Area of Controversy', Wounds, 15(5), pp. 149–66 (2003): https://miami.pure.elsevier.com/en/publications/antiseptics-on-wounds-an-area-of-controversy

20 Liikkanen, L., 'Music in Everymind: Commonality of Involuntary Musical Imagery', Proceedings of the 10th International Conference on Music Perception and Cognition, Sapporo, Japan (2008): http://l.kryptoniitti.com/lassial/files/publications/080904-Music_in_everymind_pdf.pdf

21 Liang, K.; Huang, X.; Chen, H. et al., 'Tongue Diagnosis and Treatment in Traditional Chinese Medicine for Severe Covid-19: A Case Report', Annals of Palliative Medicine, 9(4), pp. 2400–7 (July 2020). DOI: 10.21037/apm-20-1330

22 Smith, S. M.; Schroeder, K.; Fahey, T., 'Over-the-Counter (OTC) Medications for Acute Cough in Children and Adults in Community Settings', Cochrane Database of Systematic Reviews, Issue 11, art. no: CD001831 (2014). DOI: 10.1002/14651858.CD001831.pub5

23 Scharfman, B. E.; Techet, A. H.; Bush, J. W. M. et al., 'Visualization of Sneeze Ejecta: Steps of Fluid Fragmentation Leading to Respiratory Droplets', Experiments in Fluids, 57, p. 24 (2016). DOI: 10.1007/s00348-015-2078-4

24 Bhutta, M. F.; Maxwell, H., 'Sneezing Induced by Sexual Ideation or Orgasm: An Under-Reported Phenomenon', Journal

of the Royal Society of Medicine, 101(12), pp. 587–91 (2008). DOI: 10.1258/jrsm.2008.080262

25 Silva, M. F.; Leite, F. R. M.; Ferreira, L. B. et al., 'Estimated Prevalence of Halitosis: A Systematic Review and Meta-Regression Analysis', *Clinical Oral Investigations*, 22, pp. 47–55 (2018). DOI: 10.1007/s00784-017-2164-5

26 Beasley, D. E.; Koltz, A. M.; Lambert, J. E. et al., 'The Evolution of Stomach Acidity and Its Relevance to the Human Microbiome', *PLoS One*, 10(7), e0134116 (2015). DOI: 10.1371/journal.pone.0134116

27 Lindstrom, P. A.; Brizzee, K. R., 'Relief of Intractable Vomiting from Surgical Lesions in the Area Postrema', *Journal of Neurosurgery*, 19(3), p 228–36 (1962). DOI: 10.3171/jns.1962.19.3.0228

28 Gordon, C. M.; Roach, B. T.; Parker, W. G.; Briggs, D. E. G., 'Distinguishing Regurgitalites and Coprolites: A Case Study Using a Triassic Bromalite With Soft Tissue of the Pseudosuchian Archosaur *Revueltosaurus*', *Palaios*, 35(3), pp. 111–21 (2020). DOI: 10.2110/palo.2019.099

29 Horn, C. C.; Kimball, B. A.; Wang, H. et al., 'Why Can't Rodents Vomit? A Comparative Behavioral, Anatomical, and Physiological Study', *PLoS One*, 8(4), e60537 (2013). DOI: 10.1371/journal.pone.0060537

30 Gaythorpe, K. A. M.; Trotter, C. L.; Lopman, B. et al., 'Norovirus Transmission Dynamics: A Modelling Review', *Epidemiology and Infection*, 146(2), pp. 147–58 (2018). DOI: 10.1017/S0950268817002692

31 Stossel, Scott, 'Surviving Anxiety', *The Atlantic* (Jan/Feb 2014): https://www.theatlantic.com/magazine/archive/2014/01/surviving_anxiety/355741/

32 Marks, P.; Vipond, I.; Carlisle, D. et al., 'Evidence for Airborne Transmission of Norwalk-like Virus (NLV) in a Hotel Restaurant', *Epidemiology and Infection*, 124(3), pp. 481–7 (2000). DOI: 10.1017/S0950268899003805

33 Schive, K., 'Public Toilets and "Toilet Plumes"', *MIT Medical* (15 June 2020): https://medical.mit.edu/covid-19-updates/2020/06/public-toilets-and-toilet-plumes

34 Vonnegut, K., *Galapagos*, Fourth Estate (1985)

35 Spiegel, J. S., 'Why Flatulence is Funny', *Think*, 12(35), pp. 15–24 (Autumn 2013). DOI: 10.1017/S1477175613000158

36 Tomlin, J.; Lowis, C.; Read, N. W., 'Investigation of Normal

Flatus Production in Healthy Volunteers', *Gut*, 32(6), pp. 665–9 (June 1991). DOI: 10.1136/gut.32.6.665

37 Sotoudegan, F.; Daniali, M.; Hassani, S. et al., 'Reappraisal of Probiotics' Safety in Human', *Food and Chemical Toxicology*, 129, pp. 22–9 (July 2019). DOI: 10.1016/j.fct.2019.04.032

38 Lewis, S. J.; Heaton, K. W., 'Stool Form Scale as a Useful Guide to Intestinal Transit Time', *Scandinavian Journal of Gastroenterology*, 32(9), pp. 920–4 (Sep 1997). DOI: 10.3109/00365529709011203. PMID: 9299672

39 Thomson, H., 'The Anal Cushions – A Fresh Concept in Diagnosis', *Postgraduate Medical Journal*, 55, pp. 403–5 (June 1979). DOI: 10.1136/pgmj.55.644.403

40 Andrewes, C. H., 'The Natural History of the Common Cold', *The Lancet*, 253(6541), pp. 71–5 (8 January 1949). DOI: 10.1016/S0140-6736(49)90398-0

41 Centers for Disease Control and Prevention, 'Estimated Influenza Illnesses, Medical Visits, Hospitalizations, and Deaths in the United States: 2019–2020': https://www.cdc.gov/flu/about/burden/2019-2020.html

42 van Driel, M. L.; Scheire, S.; Deckx, L. et al., 'What Treatments Are Effective for Common Cold in Adults and Children?', *British Medical Journal*, 363: k3786 (10 October 2018). DOI: 10.1136/bmj.k3786

43 https://clinicaltrials.gov/ct2/show/NCT00822575

44 Wood, C.; Harrison, G.: Doré, C. et al., 'Selective Feeding of *Anopheles gambiae* According to ABO Blood Group Status', *Nature*, 239(165), p. 165 (1972). DOI: 10.1038/239165a0

45 Mellanby, K., 'Man's Reaction to Mosquito Bites', *Nature*, 158(554), pp. 912–13 (1946). DOI: 10.1038/158554c0

46 Schmidt, J., *The Sting of the Wild*, Johns Hopkins University Press (2016)

47 Season 4, episode 1

48 https://www.penguin.co.uk/articles/2019/nov/best-literary-hangovers-from-authors-and-books/

49 Nutt, D. J.; King, L. A.; Phillips, L. D., 'Drug Harms in the UK: A Multicriteria Decision Analysis', *The Lancet*, 376(9752), pp. 1558–65 (2010). DOI: 10.1016/S0140-6736(10)61462-6

50 Penning, R.; McKinney, A; Verster, J. C., 'Alcohol Hangover Symptoms and Their Contribution to the Overall Hangover Severity', *Alcohol and Alcoholism* 47(3), pp. 248–52 (2012). DOI: 10.1093/alcalc/ags029

51 Kowalski, K. and Clark, E., 'Does Mixing Drinks, Your Age or Quantity and Type of Alcohol Make for a Worse Hangover?', Society for the Study of Addiction (22 Sep 2020): https://www.addiction-ssa.org/does-your-age-drink-type-mixing-drinks-and-quantity-make-for-worse-hangovers/

52 Klostranec, J. M.; Vucevic, D.; Crawley, A. P. et al., 'Accelerated Ethanol Elimination Via the Lungs', *Scientific Reports*, 10, p. 19249 (2020). DOI: 10.1038/s41598-020-76233-9

53 Capps, R. B., 'Cause of the So-Called Side Ache That Occurs in Normal Persons: Personal Observations', *Archives of Internal Medicine* (Chicago), 68(1), pp. 94–101 (1941). DOI: 10.1001/archinte.1941.00200070104006

54 McCrory, P. A., 'Stitch in Time', *British Journal of Sports Medicine*, 41, p. 125 (2007): https://bjsm.bmj.com/content/41/3/125

55 Bell, A. I., 'Some Observations on the Role of the Scrotal Sac and Testicles', *Journal of the American Psychoanalytic Association*, 9(2), pp. 261–86 (1961). DOI: 10.1177/000306516100900202

56 Puvabanditsin, P.; Vongtongsri, R., 'Efficacy of Aloe Vera Cream in Prevention and Treatment of Sunburn and Suntan', *Journal of the Medical Association of Thailand*, 88, Suppl. 4, pp. S173–6 (2005). PMID: 16623024

57 Valtin, H., '"Drink at least eight glasses of water a day." Really? Is there scientific evidence for "8 × 8"?', *American Journal of Physiology – Regulatory, Integrative and Comparative Physiology*, 283, pp. R993–R1004 (8 August 2002). DOI: 10.1152/ajpregu.00365.2002

58 Campbell, D., 'Home Is Where the Greatest Accident Risk Is, Warns Top A&E Doctor', *Guardian* (12 Dec 2004): https://www.theguardian.com/society/2014/dec/12/home-accident-risk-nhs-doctor

59 Jonasson, F., 'Swimming Goggles Causing Severe Eye Injuries', *British Medical Journal*, 1(6065), p. 881 (2 April 1977). DOI: 10.1136/bmj.1.6065.881

60 Hall, T., 'Gardening Injuries', *Clinical Medicine Journal*, 18(5), p. 440 (Oct 2018). DOI: 10.7861/clinmedicine.18-5-440a

Index

thalamus 7
thermal injuries 113–16
Thomson, Hamish 215
throat
    glandular fever 249
    sore throat 160–1
throbbing 8
thrush 256
thunderclap headache 10
ticks 267–8
Tiger Balm 12
tineas 253–6
tinnitus 141–4
toenails, ingrowing 29, 107
toes 27
    stubbed 29
tongues 153–4
    and halitosis 175
tonsillitis 155–9
toothache 19, 45–8
torticollis 24
trapezius 24
trapped nerves 38
trapped wind 204
trench fever 275
trench mouth 176
trichomes 287
Trichosporon 256
trigeminal autonomic cephalalgias
    (TACs) 9–10
trigger points 19–22
Trowell, Hubert Carey 217
Trump, Donald J. 28
tubal tonsils 156
twitchy eyelids 105–6

ulcers
    gastric ulcers 190
    mouth ulcers 150–2
ulnar nerve 25
upper respiratory tract infections
    (URTIs) 162, 231
    and lymph nodes 234–5
    see also colds
uric acid 40
urinary tract infections (UTIs) 257
urticaria 287–8
urushiol 288–9

UVA (ultraviolet A) 310, 311
UVB (ultraviolet B) 309–10, 311
uvula 184

Valtin, Heinz 313
varicella-zoster virus (VZV) 244–5, 247
varicose veins 70, 119–21
verrucas 53, 54, 55
vestibular neuritis 139–40
Vincent's infection 176
viruses 54
Vitamin D 230
Viz 216, 315
vomiting 192–200
    and alcohol 296
Vonnegut, Kurt 201, 311

Wakefield, Andrew 243
Waldeyer's lymphatic ring 156
Wallace, Alfred Russel 287
Wallace & Gromit 140
Warren, Robin 190
warts 52–8
wasp stings 276–8
water 313, 314
water fluoridation 47–8
waxy complexion 124–5
'We Built This City' (Starship) 141, 144
Werner disease 275
wheeziness 231–2
white piedra 256
whiteheads 60, 61–2
Whitfield, Arthur 255
whitlows 251
Wight, James 308
wind
    being winded 305
    trapped 204
winter vomiting bug 194
wisdom teeth 48
worms 282–5
wound healing 88–92
wry neck 23–4

Zeis, Eduard 102
zits 60–5
    styes 102
zoster 244